FAST.
FEAST.
REPEAT.

THE COMPREHENSIVE GUIDE TO
DELAY, DON'T DENY® INTERMITTENT FASTING—
INCLUDING THE 28-DAY FAST START

Gin Stephens

ST. MARTIN'S GRIFFIN
NEW YORK

First published in the United States by St. Martin's Griffin, an imprint of St. Martin's Publishing Group

FAST. FEAST. REPEAT. Copyright © 2020 by Virginia Stephens. All rights reserved. Printed in the United States of America. For information, address St. Martin's Publishing Group, 120 Broadway, New York, NY 10271.

www.stmartins.com

The Library of Congress Cataloging-in-Publication Data is available upon request.

ISBN 978-1-250-75762-3 (trade paperback)
ISBN 978-1-250-62448-2 (ebook)

Our books may be purchased in bulk for promotional, educational, or business use. Please contact your local bookseller or the Macmillan Corporate and Premium Sales Department at 1-800-221-7945, extension 5442, or by email at MacmillanSpecialMarkets@macmillan.com.

First Edition: 2020

10 9

This book is dedicated to you,
the intermittent fasters of the world,
whether you're new to IF or a seasoned IFer.

To you, newcomers: Welcome to freedom! Consider this book a valuable resource as your IF practice progresses over time. Read and reread! Some of the information in these pages won't click until the second, third, or fourth reading. You see, as you become an experienced IFer, you'll understand things differently, including concepts that may not have made sense the first time. Promise me that you'll keep coming back to these pages from time to time. In many ways, you won't recognize yourself in a year!

To all experienced IFers, particularly readers of my first book, **Delay, Don't Deny:** I want this book to be your go-to source for all things IF! This new book is a deeper dive into the science, and my goal is for you to read it and think, *I didn't know that!* as you go along. It's true: I'm still learning things every day, even though I have years of IF under my belt.

And for all of you, whether new to IF or a seasoned IFer:
My wish is that intermittent fasting will free you from diets forever
as you learn to delay rather than deny.

ALSO BY GIN STEPHENS

Delay, Don't Deny

Delay, Don't Deny: Digging Deeper

Delay, Don't Deny: Life Journal

Feast Without Fear

CONTENTS

FOREWORD

"Thank you for telling me about Delay, Don't Deny intermittent fasting! It is truly life changing!"

In my nearly twenty years as a primary care physician, I've heard similar enthusiasm on occasion, but since I've been advocating for intermittent *fasting*—specifically Gin Stephens' *Delay, Don't Deny: Living an Intermittent Fasting Lifestyle*—I hear this kind of excitement regularly. Recommending Gin's first book has been the single most effective intervention that I, as a primary care physician, have ever made. In my patients' experiences, it has been more effective than any medication, program, or diet. It has also become a lifestyle for me, one that has allowed me to lose weight, have more energy, and—in an amazing non-scale victory—erased all joint pain. IF is an exceptionally livable, flexible lifestyle. I have done it while at home and also while I have traveled and celebrated: truly FEASTING and Fasting. I have lived this lifestyle for almost two years now, and have no intention of ever going back to "three squares and snacks"!

Gin has done it again—building on the science that she presented in her first book, and continuing to instruct readers about how to make Intermittent Fasting a *livable* lifestyle! *Fast. Feast. Repeat.* is a highly informative, readable guide to both the science behind intermittent fasting and the methods and tricks that make an intermittent fasting lifestyle both practical and easy. She presents the complex scientific concepts—like the teacher she is—by breaking them down in a way that is very easy to understand. You may even feel like you're having a discussion with Gin when you read this book: her writing style is so warm and personal and conversational.

Gin's 28-day FAST start is the perfect way to ease into and adjust the fast/feast pattern—letting your body begin to heal and become good at tapping into its fat stores. Her Clean Fast Challenge will convince you that clean fasting is the key to making IF a lifestyle and not a diet. In *Fast. Feast. Repeat.* you'll find new information, clear instruction on clean fasting, and more in-depth descriptions of styles of fasting—including alternate-day fasting, 18:6, 19:5, OMAD and others—than she's ever delivered before.

In December 2019, the *New England Journal of Medicine* published a review article about the many health benefits of intermittent fasting that not only solidified my conviction about its benefits, but was very specific in its declaration that IF is NOT just about calorie restriction: "the benefits of IF are dissociated from its effects on weight loss. These benefits include improvements in glucose regulation, blood pressure, and heart rate; the efficacy of endurance training; and abdominal fat loss." In everyday language, this means that while we often come to IF for weight loss, we remain intermittent fasters for the broad health benefits: lowering blood pressure, reducing risk of diabetes/improving diabetes and reducing abdominal fat, the accumulation of which has long been known to be detrimental for health. The article goes on to mention the benefits related to neurodegenerative disorders, cancer risk reduction, longevity, dyslipidemia, insulin resistance, and inflammation. This means that IF *is* the "magic pill." It is what we've all been looking for. For the first time in my professional life, I've been able to regularly de-prescribe medications for my patients. It is no longer unusual to lower or eliminate a patient's blood pressure medication or diabetes medication or cholesterol medication. If the pharmaceutical or diet industry could do any single one of these things consistently, it'd be a home run in terms of sales and profit. Fortunately for us, Intermittent Fasting is *free*, and it can do all of these things, not just one!

If you are just curious or ready to dive in with your very first fast— or if you've been a longtime faster—you will find a great resource in *Fast. Feast. Repeat.* What are you waiting for? Join the health revolution!

—Julie Sandell, DO,
Family Medicine Physician,
Cedar Falls, Iowa

WELCOME TO THE REST OF YOUR LIFE!

Hi, y'all! My name is Gin Stephens, and I'm so glad you have picked up my book! This is a very exciting day, because you are ready to finally get off the diet roller coaster and begin living your life on your own terms. While I will present you with information about a remarkable health and wellness strategy called *intermittent fasting* in the pages of this book, the whole time you are reading, I want you to remember that *you* are in charge, not me. *You* get to choose what you eat and when you eat it. *You* are the expert on your own body, and *today is the day* that you take back your own power. We've given away control for too long, following "expert" meal plans and protocols. This time, it's different. Together, we will work to craft the right plan for your body, and you will learn how to tweak and make changes that are just right for you.

Let me introduce myself. Who am I, and how did I come to write this book? Let's talk about my qualifications. I want you to know who I am and, most important, who I am not.

I have a bachelor's degree in elementary education, a master's degree in natural sciences, and a doctorate in gifted education. I am a teacher who has been trained to develop curriculum and present information to others. I have a broad scientific knowledge base, and I have also studied research methodologies. I can read and interpret scientific studies, make sense of them, and then redeliver the content in a way that others can understand. Because I taught elementary school for twenty-eight years, I have the heart of a teacher. Because I worked with gifted learners, I am a questioner. Because I have a science and research background, I understand both the strengths and limitations of scientific studies.

Here's who I am not: I am not a medical professional, I am not a nutritionist, and I am not a laboratory researcher. So, as you read my words, feel free to double-check everything I am saying by going straight to the studies and source material that I reference. I pledge that I am not going to misrepresent any of the scientific material that I present like so many authors do. (This is actually a real problem with many books in the health field. More times than I can count, I have read a claim and then gone to the study referenced by the author, and it's like we were reading two different papers: the original study doesn't say what the book author claims it says. I promise not to do that to you.)

I wrote my first book, *Delay, Don't Deny: Living an Intermittent Fasting Lifestyle* in 2016. After losing over eighty pounds and keeping the weight off, I wanted to share what I knew about intermittent fasting with the world, and *Delay, Don't Deny* helped me do that. I'm really proud of that book, which has been a number one bestseller on Amazon in the weight-loss category. That little book brought tens of thousands of readers to intermittent fasting, which is thrilling. Now, however, it's time for an updated book with updated advice based on the latest research. I am excited to share all of this with you here in *Fast. Feast. Repeat.* I'm also going to take a much deeper look at the science than I did in *Delay, Don't Deny,* so if you read my first book, you will still learn a lot of new things here.

I am also the host of a couple of top-rated intermittent fasting podcasts. Listen to *The Intermittent Fasting Podcast* if you want to hear us answer listener questions on a wide variety of fasting-related topics, and if you want to be inspired, listen to *Intermittent Fasting Stories,* where I talk to a cross section of real-life intermittent fasters from around the world who share both their struggles and their celebrations.

My experience has taught me a lot about intermittent fasting and the challenges faced by real people who are living an intermittent fasting lifestyle. I started a small online support group back in 2015 that has grown into several different online support groups with hundreds of thousands of members from all seven continents. (Yes, we finally have a member stationed in Antarctica!) I have spent several years mentoring and supporting our group members, and so I have a great deal of practical experience with helping others create just the right intermittent fasting lifestyle for them. I know the questions people ask, and I know the common pitfalls. I know what tweaks to try when you are struggling, and I have just the right amount of tough love that you may need to hear: intermittent fasting may be simple, but it isn't always easy! I will share all my knowledge here in *Fast. Feast. Repeat.* to help you craft your own intermittent fasting lifestyle.

So, now you know about my qualifications. You may still wonder: In what ways am I just like you? What do I know personally about diets and the struggles related to weight management?

Like many of you, I spent most of my adult life obsessed with food, dieting, and my weight. After watching my mother struggle with her own weight for most of my childhood and teen years, I internalized that this is just what we do: we go on diets, we criticize our bodies, and we are either being "good" or being "bad" with every bite we take (or don't take). Of course, it's not my mother's fault, because this obsession is everywhere we turn. You can't scroll through your newsfeed without seeing ads for *AMAZING!* weight-loss products. You can't go to the grocery store without seeing the tabloids proclaiming: *DROP 3 DRESS SIZES BY NEXT TUESDAY WITH THIS SECRET HERB FROM THE RAIN FOREST!* You can't get together with friends without discussing the latest *MIRACLE DIET!* that your most enthusiastic friend is on, where he eats nothing but foods harvested by the light of the moon. Yep. We are bombarded by "amazing" and "miracle" diets from every angle. If we could just find that magical plan or supplement or herb, the struggle would be over, once and for all. But we never do, so we keep bouncing from diet to diet and plan to plan. And we have a junk drawer full of those expensive products that we can't bear to throw away, because one day we might want to try them again, and maybe they will work this time.

Sure, we can lose some weight with those plans. I always got off to a spectacular start, which fizzled out pretty quickly when I got tired of following the restriction du jour. I was only able to white-knuckle it through the counting (calories, points, fat grams, net carbs) or prepping (buying expensive specialty foods that matched my blood type or fit the criteria of my new plan) for a limited amount of time. I have great respect for anyone who can keep this up long term, but I could not. Sound familiar?

I longed for the freedom of being able to eat delicious foods without doing a math problem first to calculate whether they fit into my plan. I didn't want to count the number of crackers I was eating or weigh out a tiny portion of cheese. Or, worse yet, avoid the crackers (if I was low-carbing it) or skip the cheese (if the diet book I was reading said that dairy was off limits). I wanted to eat cheese and crackers together, with no stress or angst.

Thank goodness for intermittent fasting. Now, I can do just that. I can have a serving of cheese and crackers and stop when I have had enough. I don't need to eat them in secret (because everyone knows that calories you eat in secret don't count, right?). I don't need to worry that I'm doing something wrong or "ruining my diet" when I eat a celebratory meal with friends. Now, I simply eat the foods that are delicious and make me feel great, and I stop when I am satisfied. Intermittent fasting has given me the freedom to completely stop stressing about food and dieting, once and for all.

Are you ready to get started? I don't blame you! Freedom awaits! Turn the page and get ready to change your life.

Are you extra-eager to get started? Ha! I get that, too. Go straight to the FAST Start section on page 116 and start there . . . but first, promise me you will come back to the beginning and read the whole book afterward. I am a teacher, and just as I always knew when a student didn't have his homework, I will know it if you don't. #TeachersSeeAll

INTRODUCTION:
THE DISMAL TRUTH ABOUT DIETS

You may have heard a surprising statistic—it's often said that about 95 percent of those who lose a significant amount of weight regain most of it. Or they may even go on to gain *more* weight, and they end up heavier than when they'd started. While there is some debate as to whether this statistic is accurate or not, we do know that the weight-loss industry in the United States was worth *$66 billion* in 2017. If diets worked long term, we wouldn't keep throwing so much money at the problem, would we? (I have some good news for you here—intermittent fasting is **free**, it requires **no** supplements, and it might even save you money in the long run, since you won't be eating as frequently.)

Why is it so hard to lose weight and keep it off? It's because of our hormones and metabolic processes. Anyone who has had this struggle has felt the way our bodies seem to fight against us over time, leaving us heavier and worse off metabolically than we were before. The good news is that it isn't your fault, and it isn't because you are weak or can't control yourself. It's biology.

Let's take some time to go down what I like to call the *memory lane of dieting.* Or you could call it *Diet Crazy-Town.* I think most of us have been there, either as a visitor or a permanent resident.

When I first jumped on the diet roller coaster, it was the 1980s and calories were king. It didn't matter what you ate, just how many calories you consumed. I carried around my pocket-sized calorie counter and my little notebook and recorded every morsel that crossed my lips. Because I was young, I was always able to lose weight as long as I kept to 1,200 calories or fewer per day. Eventually, this strategy stopped working for me, and you will understand why as you continue to read this chapter. Even though it seemed to work for me at the time, it was no fun at all to put that much thought into what I was eating (*Did I eat three chips, or four?*), so I would get to my goal weight and then abandon calorie counting completely until my weight rebounded back up, and out came the notebook once again. What a vicious cycle to be trapped in!

Next up: the low-fat era! It was the 1990s, and fat was the villain. I read my first diet book, *The T-Factor Diet,* and it all made so much sense! America agreed; this decade marked the proliferation of fat-free products. Breakfast could consist of a fat-free muffin washed down with a Coke (because Coke is fat-free!). I remember making my favorite sandwich of the time: fat-free bologna on fat-free bread, spread with fat-free mayo and fat-free mustard. Sometimes I would have a whole sleeve of those fat-free marshmallow cookies covered in fat-free chocolate. Remember how fat-free cheese wouldn't really melt, but instead looked like a square of orange plastic? Good times. (Funny story: I found a used copy of *The T-Factor Diet* recently and reread it. It's actually all about choosing real foods that happen to be lower in fat, such as vegetables, whole grains, fruits, and lean meats. Nowhere in the plan did the author recommend that you buy Franken-products as fat substitutes. Oops. Somehow, we all missed that part.) I did lose weight as long as I kept my fat grams below a certain threshold, but when I look at photos of myself from that era, I looked very thin and yet completely unhealthy. Of course I did; I don't think I was actually eating any *real* food in my quest to find fat-free food-like products.

After that, America turned against carbs. The low-fat crowd had it all wrong, and it was *carbs* we should be avoiding. During that phase, Dr. Atkins was my guru, as well as the Hellers, who determined that we were all "carbohydrate addicts" and told us what to do in *The Carbohydrate Addict's Diet.* Once again, I started counting, and I ate as much as I wanted of the allowed low-carb foods. I never did lose any weight on a low-carb plan (which I now understand after having my DNA analyzed: according to my genetic profile, I am more likely to lose weight with a higher-carb/lower-fat approach. More about that in another chapter!). Everywhere we turned, there were low-carb versions of our favorite foods and plenty of Franken-food carb substitutes.

Of course, those are just a few of the diets I tried. In addition to the big diet trends of the decades, I jumped on every bandwagon that came along: I ate right for my blood type; I counted bites as if I had gone through weight-loss surgery (yes, this is a real diet plan, and yes, I can take really big bites); I ordered tasteless, expensive, and unappealing food through the mail; I tried hypnosis; I ate "clean"; I ate "dirty"; I used costly meal replacement shakes (and even tried to sell them to my friends to support my habit); I sweated to the oldies; and more. I even went through some physician-assisted programs that included both prescription diet pills and hormone injections that tricked my body into thinking I was pregnant so I could tap into my stored fat. (I am almost embarrassed to admit the last two, but I want to keep it real . . . plus, this shows you how desperate I was. Can you relate?) Yes, those all worked temporarily, but each of them left me with more rebound weight gain than the time before. Eventually, I yo-yoed myself up to 210 pounds, which is in the obese category for my five-foot-five frame.

When I look at all the things I tried over the years, I realize that I not only lived in Diet Crazy-Town, I could have been the mayor.

Fast-forward to the present. I am maintaining a weight loss of over eighty pounds, and I haven't struggled to maintain the loss. Every year when the seasons change, I pull out my clothes from last year and try them on. I hold my breath . . . do they still fit?

And year after year, the answer is yes! Other than a few items that are now too *big*, my clothes continue to fit me season after season. I am effortlessly maintaining my weight without dieting, thanks to intermittent fasting and the magic of the clean fast, coupled with something called *appetite correction*, which you will learn about in another chapter. Instead of shopping in the plus-size department, I now fit into a size 0 or 2, and frequently I find my clothes in the petite section of the store. As the years go by and I enter my fifties (and go through menopause, with no resulting weight gain of any sort), I become more and more confident that my now-steady weight illustrates I have ended my weight struggle forever. #ThankYouIntermittentFasting

When you read my diet history, it may remind you of your own similar struggle. Yes, I am a real person, just like you. For decades, I tried and tried, and then I tried some more. If sheer effort made you thin, it would have solved the problem much earlier. If you are someone like me, you can relate to the struggle of continuing to get heavier and heavier over time, despite frantically following all the dietary advice that comes our way.

Take a deep breath.

It's time for you to realize the number one most important concept of this whole chapter: **YOU** DID NOT FAIL **DIETS. DIETS** FAILED **YOU.**

Let that sink in.

IT IS **NOT** YOUR FAULT. It's biology.

So? Why do diets like these leave us heavier and heavier over time? Why can't we succeed, even though we are trying and trying?

Heck, I would like to let you know the sad truth: the harder you *try,* the harder it *actually gets.* Again, this is biology, and *not* personal weakness or failure. In a 2013 scientific review, it was reported that in fifteen out of the twenty studies they examined, past dieting was a predictor of future weight gain.[1] That's not a surprise to all the weary dieters of the world, is it? We diet. We regain the weight. We diet again. We regain the weight again. Is it because we are gluttons? No. (Even though the "naturally skinny" people may think that's true. I remember back when I was struggling *so hard* for all the years before IF that I wanted to throttle my slim husband when he told me, "Just eat less food. Exercise more." Gee, thanks, honey. Sigh.)

No, it's not as simple as "Just eat less food. Exercise more." There are many things that go on behind the scenes in the bodies of chronic dieters that explain the phenomenon of weight gain after dieting. Let's look at the science to see why this happens.

To put it into simple terms, our bodies want us to survive and reproduce. And because of that, we have protective mechanisms that are in place to keep us from dying if our bodies perceive we are in a starvation crisis of some sort. This kept our ancestors alive during wars, droughts, and hard winters. Our bodies don't understand that we are trying to slim down for summer bathing suit season, and instead, they think we are in terrible danger.

We have a great deal of scientific research that explains how this happens in the body. Some of the earliest research on this phenomenon began in 1944. As World War II came to an end, a scientist named Ancel Keys wanted to take a close look at how the human body responded to extreme deprivation and the subsequent reintroduction of food. He and his colleagues from the University of Minnesota conducted a famous study now known as the Minnesota Starvation Experiment.[2] The topic was of immense interest because they knew that war-torn Europe faced the huge task of refeeding a population who had undergone a period of extreme deprivation due to the war. Prior to this experiment, little was known about the physiological and psychological effects of starvation. So, the purpose of this study was to gain insight into the physical and emotional effects of semi-starvation and to see what would happen when food once again became available.

Keys and his colleagues gathered thirty-six volunteers. These were young men known as *conscientious objectors,* who rejected the notion of fighting in the war but still wanted to make a meaningful contribution in a nonviolent way. For the researchers to gather baseline data, the men first went through a three-month period where they received approximately 3,200 calories of food per day, which was designed to keep their weight stable. Then they went through a six-month period where they were fed a "starvation diet" that included the foods available to the population in Europe after the war, such as potatoes and other root vegetables, brown bread, and macaroni. During the final three months, the subjects went through a "nutritional rehabilitation period" where they were randomly assigned to four different groups for a variety of refeeding methods so the researchers could determine how their bodies responded to the re-introduction of food.

During the starvation period, the expectation was for the men to lose about 2.5 pounds per week, so their food intake was decreased according to how well they were progressing toward their goals. If their weight loss slowed, the amount they were given to eat was decreased so that they would continue losing weight at the required pace. They were also expected to walk twenty-two miles per week. This certainly sounds like modern-day eat less / move more advice, am I right? If you've ever counted calories as a part of a diet plan, I am sure you remember that you had to eat less and less over time just to keep seeing weight loss, and that is just what happened here with these men.

During this starvation period, the men lost enthusiasm for their low-calorie diet as time passed. They reported having less energy, increased irritability, a decreased tolerance of the cold, and a lack of concentration. They became preoccupied with food and developed routines such as playing with their food and chewing and eating very slowly to make their meals last longer. Several of the men began collecting cookbooks and recipes, and they would spend their spare time fantasizing about food. Physically, their metabolic rates slowed over time as their calorie intake went down. They didn't just lose fat; they also lost valuable muscle mass.

Notice that Keys used the word *starvation* to refer to this period of the experiment. Every time I read about this study, it is surprising to realize that the men were fed an average of 1,800 calories of food per day during the period that was the "starvation" period. If you are a long-term dieter like me, you may look at that number—1,800—and think, *WHAT?!?!?! Seriously, 1,800 calories per day was considered starvation level?!?!?!* I remember my own low-calorie dieting days, and my calorie target was always to eat 1,200 or *fewer* calories per day—1,800 seems like a feast compared to the restrictive 1,200 I'd allowed myself. That goes to show that when we follow extreme low-calorie diet plans, we are usually subjecting ourselves to even more restriction than the participants in the most extreme "starvation" experiment in history were following.

After the starvation phase, the three-month refeeding period began. We can learn important lessons from this refeeding phase. The men continued to feel tired and weak for quite some time, and they also continued to feel extreme hunger, which for many didn't even end after they were released from the experiment to go back to their regular lives. You see, their bodies responded to the starvation period by ramping up their hunger hormones, which increased their drive to eat. This is one of the protective measures our bodies have in place to encourage us to get in the amount of food our bodies think we need to recover from the terrible tragedy we must be experiencing. One participant had to have his stomach pumped due to binge eating. Another got sick after eating in a restaurant because he simply "couldn't" stop eating. Sound familiar? Have you ever restricted calories for a while and then felt like you couldn't stop bingeing afterward? Now you know that it wasn't because you were weak; it was your body's biological drive sending you "EAT NOW!" signals. It wasn't your fault at all.

Interestingly, when the amount the subjects could eat was restricted during the refeeding phase, their resting metabolic rates stayed low—having dropped during the starvation phase—and remained low due to the continued restriction. However, when they could eat as much as they wanted, their metabolic rates rapidly recovered. This illustrates that we have hope when it comes to reversing the negative metabolic adaptations that come along with low-calorie dieting. Continued restriction over time leads to a continued decrease in metabolic rate, but eating a sufficient amount of food can actually increase your metabolic rate over time. That is very good news for any of us who may worry that we have permanently damaged our metabolisms from years of dieting—it is possible to recover!

We learned a lot from the Minnesota Starvation Experiment, but let's fast-forward to the modern era. In 2016, a group of scientists came together to examine what happened when people lost a great deal of weight quickly in a famous study that is usually referred to as the Biggest Loser Study.[3] The official title of the study was *Persistent metabolic adaptation 6 years after The Biggest Loser competition,* and just from the title, you can see that the changes continued *six years* after they had competed on the show. In the study, they discovered a continuing "metabolic adaptation," meaning that the participants had a lower resting metabolic rate (RMR) than would be predicted based upon their new body sizes and ages alone. This study resulted in sensational headlines upon its release, and the tone of the articles indicated that losing weight and keeping it off was apparently a hopeless endeavor.

You see, in this study, the participants' RMRs were calculated before they started, again at the end of the thirty-week competition, and again six years later. Overall, fourteen of the contestants participated in the follow-up study. The scientists used all the data on hand to calculate what the participants' RMRs *should* have been (based on their new sizes and ages), and when they compared the expected RMRs to their actual RMRs, they discovered that even though their RMRs were as expected at the beginning of the process (before weight loss), their average RMRs (six years later) were approximately five hundred calories lower *per day* than would be expected based on their new body sizes and ages. Not only did their metabolic rates slow, but they remained slower than expected over time. Also, the participants who lost the most weight had the greatest slowing of their metabolic rates, and those who successfully maintained more of the weight loss had an *even greater* metabolic slowing than those who did not maintain their loss. The researchers were actually surprised to see that the metabolic adaptation *increased* over the six-year period for these participants.

So, why did the most successful participants experience the greatest metabolic slowdown over time? We can look back at the Minnesota Starvation Experiment data for a clue. If you remember from the Minnesota Experiment, those who were not permitted to eat according to appetite in the refeeding phase (meaning they continued to restrict their eating over time) had metabolic rates that stayed low. Applying that to *The Biggest Loser* participants, those who managed to keep the weight off by sheer determination (and continued dieting) found that their metabolic rates continued to get slower and slower over time. Yep. This illustrates the very real truth: the harder you try to keep your calories low, the lower and lower you have to go to maintain the weight loss. While it can be done, it is a difficult (and often demoralizing) way to live your life.

Have there been other studies that also report this metabolic adaptation after a period of weight loss? Yes. In fact, multiple studies support this phenomenon.[4]

So, why does this happen?

In 2017, a group of scientists reviewed the large body of available research and found that weight loss results in an "energy gap" that leads to higher ghrelin levels (ghrelin is the hunger hormone), a larger than expected decrease in leptin (leptin is the satiety hormone), a higher than predicted decrease in resting metabolic rate, a higher than expected decrease in the thermic effect of food, and larger than predicted adaptive energy-saving behaviors. This is precisely what we saw in the Biggest Loser Study.[5]

All of that was a mouthful of scientific jargon. Let's break it down. What does this mean, in layman's terms?

Basically, when you lose weight, your body responds by:

- **Increasing ghrelin, your hunger hormone.** This means that you have an increased drive to eat. It's why you find yourself arm-deep in a bag of potato chips and you just can't seem to stop eating. Your hunger hormones are driving this behavior, not your conscious brain.

- **Decreasing leptin, your satiety, or satisfaction, hormone.** This means that you eat and eat but don't feel satisfied. It's why you keep eating until your stomach hurts—you aren't getting the "you've had enough" signal that would tell you to stop eating.

- **Lowering your metabolic rate and decreasing the amount of energy that you use daily.** And this can be as much as *25 percent below* what would be predicted based on your smaller body size. This is a protective measure; never forget that your body loves you and wants you to survive! It's why you find that your energy wanes and you just don't have the drive to get off the couch to go to the gym.

Hunger goes up. Satiety/satisfaction goes down. Metabolic rate / energy expenditure decreases. All of this works in tandem to cause the weight regain that is so common for dieters.[6]

Think about this from your experience with diets. Now you understand what went on: the longer you dieted, the harder it was to stick to the diet, and it's because your body ramped up ghrelin to send you "EAT NOW!" messages. Once we understand this, we can recognize that a stronger urge over time to "EAT NOW!" is an absolute red flag that your body is in distress, and it isn't a sign that you are "weak" or "failing." It's a sign that your body is functioning exactly as it is supposed to, in fact. So, breathe a big sigh of relief and know that we *can* trust the signals our bodies are sending us. More about that in the chapter about appetite correction. (Spoiler alert: it's absolutely amazing how fasting "fixes" our appetite signals!)

Again, please understand that all of this illustrates that it is not your fault when you "fail" at a diet. Your body is adjusting your hormone levels and metabolic processes to *save your life*. Your body doesn't know that you are trying to fit into a smaller size of clothes or look better on the beach. All your body knows is that you appear to be in some sort of danger, and drastic measures need to be taken behind the scenes so you will survive. #SayThankYouToYourBody

I know that hearing about the high failure rate of diets and the metabolic adaptations and hormonal changes that occur in our bodies when we lose weight can make us want to throw up our hands and give up before we even start. Yes, it's true that to burn stored fat and lose weight, we need to eat less food than our bodies require. And it's also true that our bodies have many protective mechanisms in place that lead to rebound weight gain after a period of restriction.

The big question is: How do we eat less food *and* keep from slowing our metabolic rates? Can we prevent this dreaded adaptation and the corresponding hormonal changes that result in rebound weight gain and a damaged metabolism?

Good news! Intermittent fasting initiates *positive* hormonal and metabolic changes in our bodies that make it very different from the low-calorie diets we have done before. So, even though you may be eating less food while living an intermittent fasting lifestyle, fasting protects your body from the more detrimental effects of metabolic adaptation. (And some people even find that they can eat *more* food than they were eating before starting IF and still lose weight, thanks to these positive hormonal and metabolic changes.) Even better, your hunger and satiety hormones get back into balance, allowing you to finally feel satisfied after eating. Hunger doesn't go up and up; it actually goes *down* over time. Keep reading to learn how this happens!

PART I

FAST.

In part 1 of *Fast. Feast. Repeat.*, you'll learn the science behind intermittent fasting (How is it better than typical "diets" for weight loss? What are the health benefits? How is it linked to longevity?). Then you will learn about the most important part of the whole process: the "clean fast," and the scientific rationale behind each of the recommendations. Next, you will be introduced to different intermittent fasting patterns, learn how to mix and match to form your own IF toolbox, and then be ready to jump right in with the twenty-eight-day FAST Start, tailored to different personality styles. Finally, you will learn how to "tweak it till it's easy."

THE STAGES OF INTERMITTENT FASTING

1. I'm going to do it! Day 1!

2. What do you mean I have to drink my coffee black???

3. The headache. Oh, I'm so tired.

4. Why am I bingeing the minute my window opens???

5. It's been six weeks, and I haven't lost weight / I'm gaining weight. HELP!

6. Hey! Suddenly I'm not as hungry! I got full before I finished my dinner!

7. I have so much energy! No more slumps during the day. This is great!

8. My pants are looser, but the scale still says I haven't lost weight.

9. All of a sudden, I am down two sizes.

10. Help! I've stopped losing weight again! What am I doing wrong???

11. None of my clothes fit. I need a smaller wardrobe!

12. Suddenly I am craving vegetables more than snack foods! Who am I?

13. #FoodSnob, when only the best will do. Food must be "window-worthy"!

14. GOAL!

15. Maintenance. I'll never eat any other way again. #DDDForLife

You may notice that you cycle through some of the steps more than once, but most people seem to experience most (if not all) of these stages along the way.

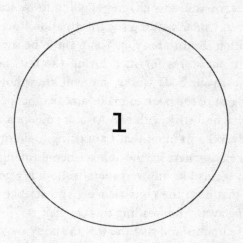

1

IGNITE YOUR FAT-BURNING SUPERPOWER!

It's true! Intermittent fasting (IF) really is different from the "eat less / move more" diets we have all tried before. One common misconception is that intermittent fasting only works because people are taking in fewer calories, making IF just another "eat less" program. (While you may find that you are eating less, we hear from many IFers that they can eat *more* calories than they were eating before beginning intermittent fasting . . . and still lose weight! Why? This chapter will explain how IF helps you tap into your fat stores like never before and also may increase your metabolic rate at the same time!)

In the introduction, I explained the science behind metabolic adaptation and how our bodies fight back when they think we are in danger of starvation. Our goal is to figure out a way to lose fat, retain our valuable muscle mass, and keep our metabolic rates from slowing down over time. Intermittent fasting is our best bet for making this happen.

I want to warn you: this chapter is going to be science-y! Don't skip it, however. Understanding the information I present here will be key in making IF work for you. You want to be sure you are tapping into your fat stores for fuel during the fast, and when you understand how your body works, you will know how to apply the lessons in the rest of the book to make sure that happens. So, put on your science hat and stick with me! Also, if you *are* a very science-y person already, keep in mind that I am going to do my best to simplify the information here for the non-science-y among us, so forgive anything that seems like an overgeneralization. My goal is to strike a balance so that both the non-science-y and science-y readers can take something away from reading this chapter.

Also, please understand that the way the body switches from one fuel source to another is incredibly complex (and actually, you're frequently using multiple fuel sources at any given moment), and so expect that my explanations are oversimplifications of the intricate metabolic processes going on within your body. I would need an entire textbook to discuss all the things that are going on behind the scenes, and it would be difficult to explain it in a way that makes sense to the layperson. Heck, some of it is even way over my head at times, even with all the time I have spent studying how this works.

Let's start with the basics. As I am sure you know, every one of us is born with the ability to store fat in times of excess and to burn that fat when times get tough. This ability kept our ancestors alive so we could all be born. The problem is that in today's era of plenty, times never do get tough, since food is all around us at every waking moment. If you work outside the home in any kind of office setting, you know what I mean—it's snack time 24-7. Even when we *do* try to diet, we seem to have lost the ability to tap into our fat stores long term, and so we yo-yo down and then right back up again. Why is this happening? How did we get into this state to begin with? And why is obesity rising at an alarming rate, even among our kids?

Let's learn about insulin and how it holds the key to our fat stores! Perhaps you have heard of insulin only through the lens of diabetes. You may know that a type 1 diabetic doesn't produce the insulin needed to survive and therefore must take insulin to literally stay alive. Before doctors understood diabetes (and before insulin had been discovered), all they knew was that someone with the disease would waste away and die, no matter how much they ate. (In a minute, you'll understand why!) The flip side of that coin is type 2 diabetes, which is becoming widespread in our modern era. Did you know that type 2 diabetes is in many ways a disease of too *much* insulin? Yep. Insulin resistance, which leads to type 2 diabetes (and is linked to obesity), is the exact opposite problem from type 1 diabetes in many ways, even though they share the same name. At the root of each condition, however, lies insulin.

Let's explore what insulin does in the body, and then you will have a lightbulb moment about why type 1 diabetics usually lose weight and type 2 diabetes is associated with weight gain.

When we eat, our bodies release *insulin* to deal with the rise in blood glucose we experience after eating (actually, just tasting food leads to something called *cephalic phase insulin release,* or CPIR. More about this in chapter 4!). Insulin is a storage hormone, so it helps our cells take in the glucose from our blood and store it temporarily in the liver and muscles (as glycogen) or, once the glycogen stores are full, the excess can be converted and stored as fat.

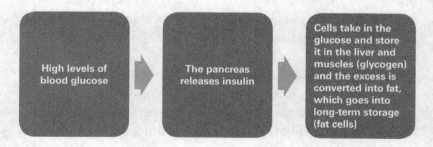

High levels of blood glucose ⟹ The pancreas releases insulin ⟹ Cells take in the glucose and store it in the liver and muscles (glycogen) and the excess is converted into fat, which goes into long-term storage (fat cells)

Over time, the levels of glucose in your blood go down (thanks, insulin, for doing your job!), and the pancreas then releases the counter-regulatory hormone *glucagon,* which signals your body to release glycogen from the liver to raise blood glucose levels so your body (and brain) can function properly. As your glycogen stores are used up, your body next starts tapping into some of the fat you've stored on your body for times like these. Your body produces ketones from your stored fat, which is a fabulous fuel for your brain in the absence of glucose.

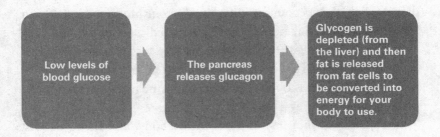

Low levels of blood glucose → The pancreas releases glucagon → Glycogen is depleted (from the liver) and then fat is released from fat cells to be converted into energy for your body to use.

This is how the body is supposed to work. We eat, our bodies release insulin, and we store the energy we don't need now for later use. We stop eating, our bodies release glucagon, and we can access the energy our bodies socked away for later. It's a beautiful thing when working properly!

Unfortunately, that is not what is happening for many of us.

The next time you are in public, look around; most people have a sweetened or flavored beverage with them at all times, and many are snacking on something throughout the day. These snacks and sweetened or flavored beverages (even the ones with zero calories) keep our bodies releasing insulin ALL. DAY. LONG. (More about this in chapter 4!)

As a result of this constant eating and drinking, many of us find ourselves in a state that can be called *hyperinsulinemia*. That is a fancy science-y word for *too much insulin*. This state of excess insulin secretion is linked to several health conditions that are plaguing our society: type 2 diabetes, metabolic syndrome, cardiovascular disease, some cancers, and Alzheimer's disease.[1]

That sounds *awful*! High levels of insulin are connected to all those health conditions? Yep.

What does this have to do with our weight? Here's a fun science word: **antilipolytic.** Let's break it down. *Anti* means *against. Lipolysis* is *fat burning.* Insulin just happens to be antilipolytic, which means that *it works against fat burning.* (If you are ever having a conversation with someone about weight loss and they start to argue with you, toss that in just to confuse them: "I was unable to lose weight in previous attempts because of high levels of insulin, which I'm sure you know is antilipolytic, Fred.")

We all know that if you want to lose weight, you must release/use more energy than you eat/store. Sounds simple, right? That's why the calories in / calories out (CI/CO) theory of weight loss makes such sense to us. On the surface, it's just math. However, when our bodies have chronically high levels of circulating insulin, we now understand that fat remains locked up in the fat cells and we can't get to it! Thank you, insulin, with your antilipolytic self.

Please understand that insulin isn't *bad*—we need it to survive! But we don't want to have too much of it, and we don't want to have high levels circulating 24-7.

Now, let's go back to the previous examples of type 1 diabetes and type 2 diabetes—have you had your lightbulb moment? Before they are diagnosed, type 1 diabetics lose weight no matter how much they eat. Why? Insufficient insulin! Their bodies are unable to clear away their excess blood glucose and store it for later! And type 2 diabetes is frequently linked to obesity. Why? Too much insulin! Their bodies are unable to easily access their fat stores for fuel, and they become locked into fat-storage mode!

In summary, we know that high levels of insulin prevent fat burning.[2] High insulin levels keep the fat virtually locked away inside your fat cells!

So why doesn't everyone design a diet plan that works with this basic fact of human biology rather than against it?

The good news is that fasting is the absolute best way to lower insulin in our bodies, bar none.[3] It is the plan that finally allows you to work *with* your body in just the way it was designed to work!

> Insulin is the key to whether your body is in fat-storing mode or fat-burning mode, and fasting puts you solidly into the fat-burning side of the equation . . . which is just what we want!

One bit of bad news that I want to share before I move on: people who are obese have *higher* fasting insulin levels and a *higher* insulin response to eating than people who are not obese.[4] This is such a vicious cycle to find yourself trapped in! If you have ever felt like you were stuck in a weight-gaining pattern and couldn't help it, now you understand why this is happening. And beyond that, besides just having chronically high fasting insulin levels, there are some factors that cause our bodies to release even more insulin! There are several known triggers, including fructose, high blood sugar levels, steroids, and certain medications.

If you are someone who has been overweight or obese for a long time, or if you are taking certain medications linked to higher levels of insulin, you may need to do more to lower your chronically high insulin levels than the average person so you can finally tap into your fat stores. More about that in chapter 22, where you'll learn what to do if weight loss is slow for you.

Now that we understand the role insulin plays in both fat storage and fat burning and that fasting helps us lower insulin, let's dig into the ways that fasting is protective of metabolic rate. In a 2016 study, scientists reported that adaptive thermogenesis (or metabolic slowdown) appeared to be related to glycogen depletion within the liver, and they speculated that the lowered metabolic rate is triggered when the brain isn't getting its energy needs met.[5]

That may have sounded complicated, but think about it this way: if you have used up your stored glycogen (meaning you no longer have access to the required amount of glucose to fuel your brain) *and* you have high insulin levels (and therefore can't tap into your fat stores efficiently for fuel), what is your body going to do for energy?

Your body needs to protect you from starving to death, and slowing your metabolic rate can keep you alive until you find the food your body thinks you need to survive (even though you have lots and lots of fuel stored on your body just for times like these).

This can be simplified as:

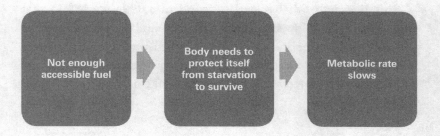

And the flip side of that:

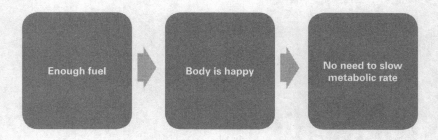

This is the key to how fasting is protective of metabolism. The body lowers insulin secretion during the fast, and insulin levels go down. Our livers release stored glycogen for energy, particularly to fuel our brains. Once we have used that energy, lowered insulin levels mean that we *can* access our fat stores and begin to break them down for fuel, creating the ketone bodies that make our brains happy by meeting their immediate energy needs. Our bodies realize we have *plenty* of stored fuel, and our metabolic rates don't slow. If, however, insulin levels remain high, we are *not* able to access our fat stores effectively, and we do *not* have access to enough fuel for our bodies (or brains).

Fasting keeps the metabolism happily chugging along, because your body realizes there is plenty of fuel!

This is exactly what scientists found in a 1994 study![6] In that study, scientists followed seventeen women and twelve men over a seventy-two-hour period of fasting and measured various changes within their bodies. There were all sorts of changes, but here are some of the most interesting ones for us to take note of:

	HOUR 12	HOUR 36	HOUR 72
Resting Metabolic Rate (RMR) (kJ/min) Higher = faster metabolic rate	4.60	4.88	4.72
Insulin levels (mU/l) Lower = less circulating insulin	≈6	≈4	≈2
Ketone levels (measured as BHB) (mmol/l) Higher = more ketones produced for energy and more fat burning occurring	≈0	≈1	≈3

We can see from the data that the subjects had an increase in their resting metabolic rates (RMR) from hour twelve to hour thirty-six of fasting, while it went back down slightly from hour thirty-six to hour seventy-two. (This is one reason why I don't recommend fasting beyond seventy-two hours: even though the RMR was still higher at seventy-two hours than it was at the twelve-hour mark, it is on a downward trend, showing that the metabolic rate is declining. We don't want to do anything that will slow our metabolic rates over time! Since this study goes to only seventy-two hours, we don't know at which point the RMR declines lower than it was when the participants started, but the downward trend should let us know it is likely to happen eventually.)

We can also see that insulin levels went down a great deal during the fasting period (Hooray! Take that, hyperinsulinemia!), and BHB (beta-hydroxybutyrate), a ketone body that provides a wonderful source of energy to our brains, went up over time. This is not the first or only study to notice that metabolic rate goes up during the first thirty-six to forty-eight hours of fasting, as several others have also found this to be true.[7]

One reason this occurs is because when fasting, our bodies are able to ignite our fat-burning superpower by "flipping the metabolic switch," a term used by a team of scientists reporting on the health benefits of fasting in a 2018 paper published in the journal *Obesity*. At what point do our bodies "flip this metabolic switch"?[8] It happens when our liver glycogen has been sufficiently depleted and fat cells are mobilized to meet our energy needs. It usually occurs at some point between hours twelve and thirty-six of fasting, and this completely depends upon how much glycogen is stored in someone's liver as well as how much energy that person is using throughout the day (as an example, exercise uses energy and helps us flip the switch sooner).

When the metabolic switch is flipped, our bodies go from running on glucose (from the foods we eat and our stored glycogen) to running on the fat from our fat cells and also the ketones that are produced to fuel our brains (and we are less likely to burn muscle tissue for fuel, since we have enough stored fat to go around and we can easily access it because insulin levels are low!).[9] Our bodies get into ketosis during the fast.

Yes, it's true. When the metabolic switch is flipped, we can produce ketones while fasting even if we are not following a ketogenic diet during our eating periods! It all has to do with the level of gly-cogen stores in our livers. Let's say someone begins IF with full liver glycogen stores, which is generally somewhere around 75–100 grams (or 300–400 calories' worth).[10] That person won't use it all up (or get into ketosis) that day, or even necessarily for the first few weeks of her intermittent fasting lifestyle. Every day, that person will deplete some of her glycogen stores during the fast. Every day, if she is fasting long enough, she depletes more than her body adds back during the eating window, even if she is eating carbs. (Not all your glucose goes into glycogen storage after you eat, by the way. Some of it is used for immediate energy needs.)

Over time, she takes out more glycogen each day than she puts back in, and through the daily fasting periods, the amount of stored liver glycogen gets lower and lower day by day. Eventually, after fasting clean for as many daily fasts as it takes her to deplete her glycogen stores sufficiently, glycogen stores are low enough that her body needs to find another fuel source for the brain. Her body switches over to fat burning, and ketosis kicks in. BOOM! The metabolic switch has been flipped! The brain is happy, because there is now a steady supply of ketones produced from stored fat.

Someone could do the same thing by doing an extended fast to burn through glycogen stores more quickly. With IF, it just takes longer to get there, because you are depleting only some of the glycogen each day. But eventually, you should get to the point where you get into ketosis daily during the fast, even while enjoying carbs in your eating window.

Our brains *love* ketones, and once we have a steady supply, we experience amazing mental clarity and increased energy during the fast! This is one of my favorite features of living an intermittent fasting lifestyle, and it is the reason that I do any work requiring me to be focused and mentally sharp while in the fasted state. (As I write this chapter, I am eighteen hours into my daily fast, so I'll likely open my eating window in the next hour or so. What do all these fasting terms mean? Don't worry! I'll explain them in chapter 6.)

Once your body has learned to tap into your fat for fuel during the fast, you have reached a state we like to call *metabolic flexibility,* and I believe it is how our bodies are meant to function. (In fact, metabolic inflexibility is linked to many of the diseases that are plaguing modern society, such as metabolic syndrome, type 2 diabetes, cancer, and other age-related diseases.)[11]

What does metabolic flexibility look like in our bodies? When we eat, we use the food for fuel. When we fast, we switch over to using our backup fuel sources for energy, including our stored fat. Voilà! Metabolic flexibility, just as nature intended! This would have been important in the past when we didn't have a grocery store or fast-food restaurant on every corner, or a pantry fully stocked with snacks. Our survival would have depended on the body's ability to switch fuel sources as needed. Regaining this flexibility is *huge.*[12]

All this talk about ketosis and ketones may make you think you need to go out and buy some of those ketone indicator strips so you can start checking your urine, a ketone breath analyzer so you can check ketones in your breath, or a blood ketone meter so you can check ketone levels in your blood. Actually, I would like to encourage you to *not* get caught up in trying to measure ketones at all.

Let me explain. When your body uses ketones efficiently, there are fewer ketones being excreted, or released, in your urine or your breath, and you also won't have as many hanging around in your blood. If you try to measure, it may appear that you are not making many ketones, when in actuality, your body is just becoming really good at *using* the ketones that you have made. If you are trying to gauge your success based on ketone readings, this could lead to frustration. Don't let this happen to you! Instead, as long as you find that you have increased energy during the fast and greater mental clarity, know that your body is doing just what it needs to do, and no measuring is required. (This won't happen on day 1! You'll need to get through the adjustment period called the FAST

Start before you experience the magic of increased energy and mental clarity.)

Now, let's talk about another important piece of the metabolic puzzle: how fasting preserves (and even increases!) muscle mass. Preserving muscle mass is important, because increased muscle mass is linked to a higher metabolic rate and also to a number of other health benefits.[13] As I've already explained, fasting allows us to preferentially tap into fat stores for fuel, because we have lowered insulin levels while fasting. Instead of being in an antilipolytic state, we have actual lipolysis! (Hooray for fat burning!) This helps to preserve our muscle mass, as our bodies wouldn't dream of using up our valuable muscle mass for fuel when there is plenty of accessible fat stored on our bodies for that very purpose.

On the flip side, if you are following a standard low-calorie diet and eating frequently during the day, your body releases insulin over and over in response to each eating (or drinking) experience. You can't tap into your fat stores very efficiently due to the high levels of insulin, and so your body is going to use whatever it can find for fuel, and that may include some of your muscle tissue. This is why you might actually lose "weight" more quickly on a traditional low-calorie diet than when following an intermittent fasting lifestyle; it reflects the loss of muscle mass. You should understand that we don't simply want to see the scale *number* go down. We want to see actual levels of *body fat* go down, and total muscle mass should either stay the same or go up. The good news is that this is exactly what we see in intermittent fasters![14] Not only is muscle preserved, but our bodies become better at building muscle tissue.

One of the main reasons IFers are better able to build muscle tissue is because fasting leads to a natural increase in our levels of human growth hormone, or HGH. Several studies have shown this increase, which is absolutely thrilling![15,16] Thanks to IF, we don't need to inject ourselves with HGH to see increased levels of this hormone within our bodies. (Did you know that bodybuilders sometimes do this to bulk up their muscle mass? Having this happen naturally is one reason many forward-thinking bodybuilders have embraced intermittent fasting.) We build muscle naturally!

Sometimes this confuses people. They say, "But, Gin! I am not going to the gym. I am not lifting weights. How can I possibly be building muscle?"

The good news is that when you have increased levels of HGH, you are more likely to gain muscle just by actively living your life.

Think about babies and toddlers. They are building muscle tissue faster than at any other point in their lives! Yet I've never seen a baby or toddler pumping iron at the gym.

Naturally, we have the highest levels of growth hormone when we are young, since this is the time of our lives when we are actively growing, and these levels decline drastically over time. With IF, we can bring these levels back up to some degree, and even though you may not be going to the gym, you are doing other things—you may be vacuuming the floor, cutting the lawn, or hauling in the groceries. You are using your muscles throughout the day as you live your life, just as babies and toddlers do.

The news about increased HGH gets better and better, by the way! HGH not only leads to enhanced muscle growth, it is also associated with higher bone density and faster healing of wounds and injuries.[17,18,19,20]

In summary, intermittent fasting is without a doubt our fat-burning superpower. Here are the main takeaways from this chapter:

FASTING	TRADITIONAL LOW-CALORIE DIETS
• Lowers insulin levels so we can access stored fat! This is the magic of the clean fast.	• Frequent small meals throughout the day lead to frequent insulin release, keeping us from burning fat efficiently.
• Metabolic rate goes UP!	• Metabolic rate goes DOWN!
• Muscle tissue is protected (and even increases, thanks to increased human growth hormone)!	• The body uses some of our muscle tissue for fuel, since the fat is somewhat locked up and harder to access due to high insulin levels.

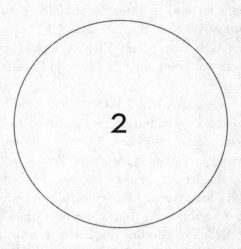

2

INTERMITTENT FASTING: THE HEALTH PLAN WITH A SIDE EFFECT OF WEIGHT LOSS

Even though intermittent fasting is our fat-burning superpower, IF is about so much more than weight loss! In fact, many of us come for the weight loss but stick around for the health benefits.

The fasting world was rocked in 2016 when Yoshinori Ohsumi won the Nobel Prize in Medicine for his groundbreaking work on autophagy, which is linked to fasting. (If the word *autophagy* is new to you, keep reading to learn more about this process that is as old as human cellular life yet still new and fresh within the science world!) Ever since then, interest in the connection between fasting and health has skyrocketed, and I can't wait to share the latest research here with you. While this chapter will be a bit science-y, just as the last one was, I will make sure to explain everything in a way that makes you just as excited as I am about the health benefits of intermittent fasting!

First, let's get one thing out of the way. A good bit of the research being conducted in the health field in general is done using animals or rodents. Some critics say that we should only discuss scientific studies done on humans, and it's true that animals and humans are different. Still, animal studies can be very useful.[1] It's a lot easier to make sure animals are compliant with the study expectations (humans, not so much!), and they can be studied in a lab in a way that it's hard to do in studies with humans. While it's easier to study animals such as mice, and they have a great many physiological similarities to humans, animal research does have limitations. Most scientists fully acknowledge that fact, even while continuing to use these animal models to study basic biological processes that we have in common. So, if you decide to dig in deeper to any of the scientific studies/research that I mention in this (or any other) chapter of the book, keep in mind both the strengths and limitations that come along with research using animals. Also keep in mind that even research using humans has flaws. Scientific research itself is complex and messy, no matter which species is being studied (which leads to a lot of the confusion and seeming contradictions we see in the health world today). Yes, much (though not all) of the research I am going to discuss may have been conducted using animal models, but that doesn't mean it doesn't have important applications for us.

One other word of caution: whenever we read flashy claims and promises related to health and wellness, it's important to understand that many of the scientific claims we see touted in books and articles may not hold up to scrutiny. As I did the research for this chapter, I spent weeks combing the scientific literature for high-quality scientific sources. My goal was to back up every claim with scientific sources that had merit. Please look at them in the reference section and read the studies themselves for more in-depth information and to confirm the claims that I am making here. And don't forget that much of the scientific understanding about the health benefits of intermittent fasting is still developing.

I have confidence that we will see more and more of this exciting research over the coming years and decades. Even though research is still ongoing, I am convinced that we are at the forefront of a health revolution!

Now that we have that out of the way, let's dig into just a few of the evidence-based health benefits of intermittent fasting! As you read, please remember that the information in this book should not be substituted for actual medical advice from your health care practitioner. Always work with your health care team to determine if intermittent fasting is right for you and if it will work with your specific health conditions.

FASTING COMBATS HYPERINSULINEMIA!

In the previous chapter, you learned that insulin is a very important hormone in the body but that too much insulin—hyperinsulinemia—is *not* a good thing. You may remember my telling you that hyperinsulinemia is linked to type 2 diabetes, metabolic syndrome, cardiovascular disease, some cancers, and Alzheimer's disease.[2]

Nothing is better at lowering our insulin levels than fasting![3] Since we release insulin in response to eating, the daily fasting time gives our bodies a break from the constant need for more insulin. One 2018 study of time-restricted feeding (within a six-hour eating window) found that the worse the participants' hyperinsulinemia was when they started, the higher the reduction in insulin levels![4] This is great news for any of us who have (or suspect we have) hyperinsulinemia! Even more great news: in a 2019 study of alternate-daily fasting where participants followed the treatment for twelve months, those in the fasting group had an average decrease of 52 percent in their fasting insulin levels (versus 14 percent in the control group) and a 52 percent decrease in their insulin resistance (versus 17 percent in the control group).[5]

FASTING CAN PREVENT AND REVERSE METABOLIC SYNDROME!

Metabolic syndrome is characterized by a cluster of symptoms, including obesity (particularly abdominal), insulin resistance, elevated triglycerides, and high blood pressure. You're probably aware that metabolic syndrome has been linked to many diseases and conditions such as an increased risk for cardiovascular disease, diabetes, stroke, and Alzheimer's disease.[6]

In studies done on rats and mice, intermittent fasting addresses each one of the defining characteristics of metabolic syndrome. When we understand that the keys to combatting metabolic syndrome include decreasing fasting glucose levels, lowering circulating levels of insulin, and reversing insulin resistance, it becomes clear how fasting would be beneficial in humans, as well.[7,8]

FASTING MAY *REVERSE* TYPE 2 DIABETES!

According to a 2019 editorial in the scientific journal *Open Heart,* "In regard to type 2 diabetes, this disorder can sometimes be *fully reversed* in its early stages if the factors that impelled its onset are corrected, that is, if a diet and exercise regimen that supports insulin sensitivity is implemented and appropriate weight loss is achieved."[9]

This is a bold statement! We have been told for years that type 2 diabetes is a chronic condition, and once you are diagnosed, all you can do is manage your condition and you should expect that your health will get progressively worse over time. Well, tell that to Dr. Jason Fung. Dr. Fung is a nephrologist from Toronto, and he works with patients at his Intensive Dietary Management clinic. He is also the author of two foundational books: *The Obesity Code* and *The Diabetes Code.* (If you or someone you love suffers from type 2 diabetes, *run,* don't walk, to get a copy of *The Diabetes Code.* You will understand type 2 diabetes in a way you never did before!)

In a 2018 case study, Dr. Fung reported the results of three of the type 2 diabetic patients who received treatment in his clinic.[10] These patients had been diagnosed as type 2 diabetics anywhere from ten to twenty-five years prior to the study period. Before beginning their fasting regimens, each patient was taking daily injections of insulin. These patients were followed for seven to eleven months, and all three of them were able to discontinue taking insulin within a *five- to eighteen-day* period after beginning their fasting protocols. All three of them lowered their A1C levels, reduced their waist circumferences, and also lost fat.

And that's not all! In a 2019 study, one week of time-restricted feeding (the eating-window approach to IF) improved glucose tolerance of men at risk for type 2 diabetes.[11] Previous studies have shown this same result (improved glucose tolerance) as well as improved insulin sensitivity in mice. A 2012 study found that patients in Utah who include fasting as a part of their religious practice had a significantly lower chance of developing type 2 diabetes.[12]

And a 2017 study of ten type 2 diabetic patients found that fasting blood glucose levels improved, as did blood glucose levels following meals.

While more clinical research is clearly needed, these results are very promising. Anecdotally, many intermittent fasters have reported similar results: lowered A1C values, medications (including insulin) reduced or eliminated completely, and even no longer being medically classified as type 2 diabetic. While these results sound incredible, we hear them all the time from intermittent fasters in our community.

One more bit of hopeful information: scientists report that intermittent fasting leads to beta cell regrowth in rodents.[13] Beta cells are the insulin-producing cells found in the pancreas. If this can be replicated in humans, then there is hope for even long-term type 2 diabetics who have suffered beta cell damage.

FASTING IS ANTI-INFLAMMATORY!

Chronic inflammation has a serious negative impact on our health. In fact, increased levels of inflammation may lead to the development of chronic conditions, such as heart disease and cancer.[14] The good news for us is that in a number of studies, intermittent fasting has been shown to improve inflammatory markers.[15,16,17]

In a 2015 study, researchers at Yale University found that BHB (beta-hydroxybutyrate), a ketone compound the body produces while fasting, is associated with this reduced inflammation.[18] In their study, they gave BHB to mice who suffered from inflammatory diseases and found that the BHB appeared to be instrumental in lowering inflammation. Remember from the last chapter that ketones are produced when you are tapping into your fat stores for fuel during the fast. So, you're not only igniting your fat-burning superpower, you're lowering your inflammation at the same time!

Several of the studies on the anti-inflammatory properties of intermittent fasting have been performed using adults fasting for Ramadan, which is a monthlong religious observance that requires Muslims to fast from dawn to sunset daily. One study found that inflammatory markers significantly decreased over the month of Ramadan.[19]

Another Ramadan study found that fasting suppressed proinflammatory molecules called *cytokines* within the body.[20] Excessive production of these types of molecules contributes to many of the inflammatory diseases so prevalent in today's society, such as allergies, asthma, autoimmune diseases, and inflammatory bowel disease, just to name a few.

In fact, in a 2008 study, patients with asthma were followed through an eight-week IF protocol, and their asthma-related symptoms decreased significantly.[21] Both their markers of oxidative stress and their indicators of inflammation went down.

On a personal note, I have had my seasonal allergies completely disappear, which is thrilling! This didn't happen overnight, by the way; I didn't see this benefit until I had consistently followed an intermittent fasting lifestyle for over two years. In case this sounds unbelievable, I have heard the same result from many intermittent fasters who are amazed to be able to stop taking allergy medications entirely. It makes sense when you understand how IF lowers inflammation!

FASTING SHOWS PROMISE FOR THOSE WITH AUTOIMMUNE DISEASES!

Autoimmune diseases, such as rheumatoid arthritis, psoriasis, multiple sclerosis, lupus, inflammatory bowel disease, and Hashimoto's thyroiditis are on the rise, particularly among women.[22] The good news is that fasting is beneficial in both preventing and controlling symptoms of many autoimmune diseases.[23] This makes sense when we understand that autoimmune diseases are closely associated with an abnormal inflammatory response; anything that lowers inflammation would tend to benefit diseases linked to increased inflammation.[24] Here is just a small sampling of some of the research into specific autoimmune diseases and fasting:

Rheumatoid arthritis: In one small study, fasting resulted in improvements in pain levels, stiffness, reliance on pain medications, and several other variables.[25] In another study, patients with RA who fasted for Ramadan exhibited reduced symptoms of morning stiffness.[26]

Psoriasis: In a 2019 study, 108 patients with moderate to severe plaque psoriasis were followed over a month of Ramadan fasting. The study found a significant decrease in the Psoriasis Area and Severity Index score.[27]

Multiple sclerosis: Our nerves are covered by a myelin sheath, and in multiple sclerosis, our bodies' own immune systems attack and destroys this sheath. This results in something called *demyelination,* which leads to an impaired transmission of nerve impulses. In a 2016 study, scientists used a "fasting mimicking diet" with mice.[28] In the study, this approach completely reversed symptoms in 20 percent of animals. They also noted a remyelination of nerve cells.

FASTING HAS CARDIOVASCULAR BENEFITS!

Heart disease is considered to be the leading cause of death around the world, and research finds that fasting has benefits related to heart health.[29] Fasting has been linked to reduced blood pressure, reduced resting heart rate, an improvement in the cardiovascular system's response to stress, and resistance of cardiac muscle to damage.[30,31]

One 2008 study showed that of 4,629 patients in Utah, those who fasted for religious reasons had a significantly lowered risk of coronary artery disease.[32] In a 2018 study, they found that time-restricted feeding (with a six-hour eating window) resulted in dramatic changes in blood pressure that equal the results typically seen through medication![33] One of the same Ramadan studies I mentioned earlier found positive effects on some of the risk factors of cardiovascular disease.[34] It's exciting to note that these were all studies done with humans.

Why is fasting so great for heart health? A 2010 study with rats gives us a clue. Scientists found increased levels of a compound called *adiponectin,* which is known to be both cardio-protective and anti-inflammatory.[35] As a result in the increase in adiponectin, the rats following the IF regimen had less systemic inflammation and reduced damage to heart cells.

FASTING IS EXCELLENT FOR BRAIN HEALTH!

If we want to age well, we know that we need to keep our brains healthy to stay mentally sharp. I want to be one of those one-hundred-plus-year-old ladies who is still going strong, both physically and mentally. I believe IF is my (not-so-secret) weapon!

Dr. Mark Mattson is a rock star in the world of fasting, and he is doing some exciting research into IF's many neurological benefits. His research shows that fasting improves neural connections in the hippocampus and protects our brains against the accumulation of amyloid plaques. Benefits of fasting include fewer signs of depression, improved memory, increased production of neurons, and an enhanced ability of our brains to ward off neurodegenerative diseases like Alzheimer's and Parkinson's.[36,37,38,39]

In the brain, IF has been shown to increase brain-derived neurotrophic factor (BDNF), improve synaptic plasticity, and improve resistance to both injury and disease.[40] One mouse study showed that IF improved both cognitive function (related to learning and memory) and the overall structure of the brain.[41] In mouse models of Alzheimer's disease, IF protected the brain against cognitive decline.[42] Because intermittent fasting decreases neural degeneration, studies show that IF results in fewer symptoms related to Alzheimer's disease, Parkinson's disease, and Huntington's disease.[43] BDNF, which I just told you is increased during fasting, helps prevent these neurodegenerative disorders by increasing the resistance of brain neurons to this degeneration. Low levels of BDNF are also associated with depression, so higher levels of BDNF would be expected to be helpful for those suffering from depression (in fact, some conventional antidepressants also raise levels of BDNF).[44] A 2013 study on mood and depression found significant mood improvements when aging men followed an intermittent fasting regimen for three months, which is just what we would expect to see if BDNF increased.[45]

FASTING DECREASES VISCERAL FAT!

We have two main types of fat: subcutaneous fat (found beneath the skin, such as the fat on your thighs) and visceral fat (found around your organs). Increased levels of visceral fat have been linked to an increased risk of health conditions such as diabetes and even increased mortality.[46] Intermittent fasting has been shown to lower both overall fat mass and this more dangerous visceral fat.[47]

In a 2016 study, scientists found that intermittent fasting led to something surprising. First, they found that our bodies prefer to burn the unhealthy visceral fat for energy first.[48] During fasting, this visceral fat is more efficient at meeting our energy needs than the subcutaneous fat. Here's where the surprise comes in: under fasting conditions, the subcutaneous fat underwent a switch to become more like the visceral fat, making it easier to access and turning it into what the scientists called a "backup energy reservoir." This is a win-win! We use up the unhealthy visceral fat *and* the stubborn subcutaneous fat!

FASTING ADJUSTS OUR HUNGER AND SATIETY HORMONES!

One of the amazing features of intermittent fasting is the way it affects our natural appetite control system. Ghrelin is known as the hunger hormone, because our bodies ramp it up to send us the signal that we need to eat. On the flip side of that, leptin is the satiety hormone, and our bodies use leptin to send us the signal that we have had enough food. We are born with fully functioning appetite control signals. Think of a baby. A hungry baby cries until it is fed. A baby that has had enough, however, stops eating and can't be coaxed to take in another drop. Somehow along the way, we lose touch with these natural signals. I'll talk more about this in the upcoming chapter about the phenomenon we call *appetite correction.*

How does fasting help? Research shows that IF decreases ghrelin (the hunger hormone) and increases leptin (the satiety hormone).[49,50] I like to think of it as a factory reset back to how we were prior to losing touch with these appetite signals. It's one of the most striking features of living an IF lifestyle, in fact!

FASTING CAN "RESET" THE GUT MICROBIOME!

Over recent years, we have learned that a healthy gut microbiome is essential for overall health. Prior to the 2000s, scientists didn't know much about what lived in that dark and rather smelly part of our bodies, but new technology in DNA sequencing has allowed for amazing discoveries over the past couple of decades.[51] Besides being the place your poop is passing through, our gut is home to *trillions* of microorganisms that make up your gut microbiome.

We now know that our gut microbiomes are an important part of our immune systems' function and also play a key role in our overall metabolic health.[52] Did you know there is a striking difference in the inhabitants of the gut microbiomes of people who are lean and people who are obese?[53] And that a fecal transplant from an obese person to a lean person (yes, I'm talking about a poop transplant) can lead to the lean person becoming overweight, with no changes in eating habits?[54]

The good news is that we can change our gut without a fecal transplant. Studies on time-restricted feeding in mice have found that fasting leads to reduced gut permeability, increases the diversity of the gut microbiome, and shifts the population to one associated with leanness rather than obesity.[55] Change your gut, change your health!

FASTING IS ANTITUMOR AND HAS POSITIVE EFFECTS DURING CANCER TREATMENT!

Fasting shows promise at both preventing tumor growth and also as a therapy that is useful as a part of a chemotherapy regimen.[56]

Some of the proposed mechanisms of fasting's anticancer benefits include:[57]

- reduced rate at which cells increase;

- a positive and low-intensity stress to the body, which leads to protective effects;

- lowered oxidative stress that can be linked to the growth of cancers;

- increased antioxidant activity; and

- increased autophagy (which I will discuss in more detail in a minute—stay tuned!)

Earlier, we learned that hyperinsulinemia can be related to tumor growth. This finding explains why certain cancers are linked to obesity (and also reminds us of how chronically elevated insulin levels are detrimental in so many ways!).[58] While we still don't have significant research findings linking fasting to cancer prevention in humans, in rats, fasting increased longevity by 15–20 percent and also reduced tumor growth by 65–90 percent.[59] Over time, we hope to see more studies that involve humans.

What if someone has already been diagnosed with cancer? When fasting is used in combination with chemotherapy, studies have shown that the cancer cells are unable to adapt and are unprotected, while the body's normal cells receive protective benefits from the fasting.[60,61,62] While I hope that my intermittent fasting lifestyle protects me from ever developing cancer, if I were ever to be diagnosed with a tumor of any kind, I would not rest until I found an oncologist who was familiar with the research into using fasting along with chemotherapy.

FASTING INCREASES AUTOPHAGY!

I told you about the ripples of excitement that ran through the intermittent fasting world in 2016 when Yoshinori Ohsumi won the

Nobel Prize in Medicine for his groundbreaking work on the process of autophagy. Suddenly, this formerly unknown word was on everyone's lips.

For the rest of this chapter, I am going to teach you about autophagy: it's one of the most exciting health benefits of all!

What is autophagy? Literally, it means *self-eating*.[63] It's an important cellular mechanism that helps our cells survive when faced with stressors like starvation.

To understand autophagy, think of it as our bodies' ultimate upcycling program. What is upcycling? According to *Wikipedia*, upcycling is "the process of transforming by-products, waste materials, useless, or unwanted products into new materials or products of better quality and environmental value."[64] That is precisely what autophagy does in the body: autophagy transforms our bodies' by-products, waste materials, useless, or unwanted products into new materials or products of better quality and environmental value!

Elementary teachers are *great* upcyclers! Somehow, we teachers are all born with the instinct to take junk and turn it into something useful. We can make comfy seating nooks out of old tires, discarded paint buckets, and milk crates we borrowed from the cafeteria. Give us your old cereal boxes and we can make board games, playing cards, and book display shelves. Just as teachers are born with the upcycling instinct, so are our bodies. Trash becomes treasure, whether we are upcycling in our classrooms or upcycling within our own bodies.

So, our bodies use the process of autophagy to recycle damaged or unwanted cell parts to use them for energy or for building blocks for new growth. Damaged organelles? Autophagy upcycles their parts! Intracellular pathogens? Autophagy to the rescue! Got cellular junk? Autophagy for the win!

When we are fasting, autophagy increases to ensure our survival in the absence of food intake.[65]

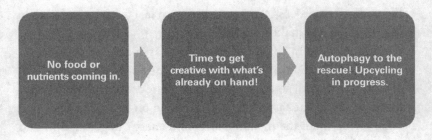

No food or nutrients coming in. → Time to get creative with what's already on hand! → Autophagy to the rescue! Upcycling in progress.

I absolutely love the thought that while I am fasting every day, my body is looking for old cellular junk to remake into a spiffy new body part.

If you've ever watched a TV show or read a magazine article where people lost massive amounts of weight, usually they are left with a great deal of excess skin. Personally, I lost over eighty pounds, and that means I need a lot less skin to cover my new slim body—yet I don't have any problematic excess skin. What happened to all that excess skin as I lost weight? Dr. Jason Fung claims that he has never had to send a patient to the plastic surgeon for skin removal surgery, even when they lose over one hundred pounds.[66] His theory is that autophagy breaks down the old skin tissue and uses it to build new body parts.

Autophagy does a lot more within our bodies than just upcycling old skin tissue, of course. Our goal is to ensure that autophagy occurs on a frequent basis, just as nature intended. When autophagy is blocked somehow within the body, this can lead to the onset of cancer, liver disease, aging, metabolic syndrome, or neurodegeneration.[67,68] I want to make sure that I am experiencing all these benefits daily.

This can cause a lot of confusion. When does autophagy happen, exactly? How can we *know* it's happening? Will we experience increased autophagy when we follow a daily intermittent fasting approach, or do we need to do extended fasts to reap these benefits?

Think about this for a minute. Would your body have an amazing cellular cleaning process that requires you to fast for days and days to access it? It doesn't make any sense, does it?

As I taught you in chapter 1, our bodies are designed to be metabolically flexible. Before the modern era, our ancestors had to hunt and gather to be fed, so they would have periods of time where they were naturally in the fasted state. They relied on ketosis to fuel their brains, giving them the mental clarity and energy to go out and find the food they needed. This metabolic flexibility would have gotten them through both the daily quest for food and the lean times.

Increased autophagy is part of this important adaptation and is linked to the state of ketosis. These processes happen when your metabolic switch is flipped and your body has to scrounge around for fuel. Think about it this way: Imagine that you haven't been to the grocery store for a long time, you're snowed in, and your fridge and pantry are fairly bare—but you're hungry! You will need to dig to see what you have lying around that you could make into a meal. This is what happens when your body is in the fasted state; your body is foraging around within for fuel (which leads to *fat-burning* and *ketosis*) and also searching for whatever building blocks can be torn down and reused (which happens through increased *autophagy*). So, while ketosis and autophagy are *not* the same process, they both occur when the body has a need to scrounge around to see what's on hand.[69,70,71]

You'll often hear someone in the intermittent fasting community say that autophagy doesn't ramp up until someone is twenty-four to thirty-six hours into the fasted state. That statement causes a lot of confusion for many people, and that's because it doesn't tell the whole story! Recall the lesson from the last chapter about getting into ketosis once we deplete our liver glycogen sufficiently to get into the fat-burning state. It's true that it might take someone twenty-four to thirty-six hours to do this (or even longer) *if they are beginning with full glycogen stores.* But remember, after our bodies become metabolically flexible, we no longer have full glycogen stores! We are able to get into ketosis daily when we are in the fasted state (this may happen at around hour twelve of the fast, though it might take as long as sixteen to twenty-plus hours, depending upon what and how much you eat, your activity level, and even how much insulin your body has circulating). And since we know that when ketosis ramps up, so does autophagy, you can be assured that you are receiving benefits from increased autophagy without having to fast regularly for twenty-four to thirty-six hours or beyond.[72]

It's true that if you fast longer, you'll get more deeply into ketosis and experience even higher levels of autophagy, but it is not required. Trust that your body will make the most of your daily fasting period, with no longer fasts required . . . unless you *want* to fast longer. More about that in chapter 7!

Now that we have learned about some of the exciting health benefits linked to intermittent fasting, it's time to learn about another thrilling discovery: intermittent fasting is linked to increased longevity! More about these exciting discoveries in the next chapter.

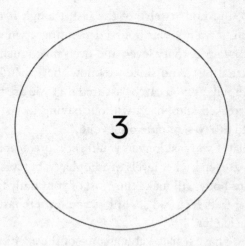

3

FASTING: THE REAL-LIFE FOUNTAIN OF YOUTH?

Not only is fasting linked to the long list of positive health outcomes that I presented in the previous chapter, scientists are also reporting that fasting comes with a host of benefits that may be linked to longevity for humans. While much of this research is being done on animals, there are some promising results from human studies, as well. In this chapter, I am going to summarize just a bit of the most cutting-edge research into the link between fasting and longevity. Make sure to visit the references section and dig into these studies for yourself if you have a deeper interest in the topics.

In 2019, scientists in Okinawa released a groundbreaking study using human subjects that found some surprising results.[1] I always love to read the titles of these studies because all the science-y words make them sound so impressive. This study is called *Diverse metabolic reactions activated during 58-hr fasting are revealed by nontargeted metabolomic analysis of human blood*. Let's dig in just a bit and see what they found!

In the Okinawan study, four volunteers participated in a fifty-eight-hour fast, and researchers took blood samples at specific intervals: at ten, thirty-four, and fifty-eight hours into the fast. (Yes, this is a small sample size. Yes, it is still exciting! The next steps will include repeating this study with a larger sample.) Does this mean that we have to fast for fifty-eight hours to get these benefits? No. Increases in all these compounds were seen between hours ten through thirty-four of the fast, as well.

Why is this study so exciting? As we age, levels of many important metabolites, which are substances produced by the body as a result of metabolic processes, decline. Seeing increased levels of these metabolites is, therefore, very exciting. Of the forty-four compounds they identified in this study, only fourteen of them had been previously associated with the fasted state. These metabolites are linked to the maintenance of muscle tissue and also antioxidant activity that can help prevent some of the damage we see related to aging. Sounds like the fountain of youth to me!

A quote from the authors:

During human fasting, metabolic markers, including butyrates, carnitines, and branched-chain amino acids, are upregulated for energy substitution through gluconeogenesis and use of stored lipids . . . we identified . . . hitherto unrecognized metabolic mechanisms induced by fasting . . . probably due to demand for antioxidants, NADPH, gluconeogenesis and anabolic metabolism . . . Global increases . . . of compounds reflect enhanced mitochondrial activity in tissues during fasting . . . Thus diverse, pronounced metabolite increases result from greatly activated catabolism and anabolism stimulated by fasting. Antioxidation may be a principal response to fasting.

Whoo. That's a mouthful, isn't it?

Let's understand what all of this means by using simpler terms. What are some of the specific things they found?

Fasting increased levels of:

- **Butyrates**

  Butyrates are short-chain fatty acids that have a whole host of positive health benefits, including (but not limited to) anti-inflammatory properties, immune system regulation, and prevention and treatment of insulin resistance.[2]

- **Carnitines and branched-chain amino acids**

  You may have heard of these as ingredients found in supplements promoted by bodybuilders. Both are often in pre- or post-workout supplements designed to aid in muscle growth. It's exciting to note that we don't need to supplement with them; our bodies can take care of our needs naturally! These compounds not only promote muscle growth, they also help reduce the breakdown of muscle cells.

- **Antioxidants**

  We have all heard of antioxidants, usually in the context of choosing foods that have high levels of these health-promoting compounds. The good news is that our bodies also produce compounds that have antioxidant properties. These compounds work in our bodies to defend cells against harmful molecules called *free radicals,* which can damage our cells (this cell damage can lead to many of the illnesses and conditions associated with aging).

- **Mitochondrial activity**

  The mitochondria are often called *the powerhouses of the cell* because they work as the "digestive system" of the cell, taking in nutrients, breaking them down, and turning them into forms of energy the cell can use. The mitochondria also serve an important role in breaking down waste products within the cells (autophagy for the win!).[3] In addition, the mitochondria are instrumental in a process called *apoptosis,* which you can think of as autophagy's bigger-and-badder cousin. In simple terms, apoptosis is "programmed cell death." While that sounds terrifying, we actually *do* want certain cells to "die," and these include infected, damaged, or other unwanted cells.[4] Fasting ramps up all these protective mitochondrial processes.

- **Catabolism**

To put it simply, *catabolism* is the breakdown of something into smaller pieces. For example, autophagy is a catabolic process that lets our bodies break down something we don't need any longer.[5] Fasting ramps up these catabolic processes.

- **Anabolism**

Anabolism is the opposite of catabolism. It's when our bodies take a bunch of pieces and put them back together in a new way. As an example, the body can take a bunch of amino acids that were broken down from old parts and use them in the process of making new muscle cells. Talk about upcycling! Old junk turned into valuable muscle tissue![6]

One thing that is especially exciting about this 2019 research out of Okinawa is that it wasn't done on rats or mice but was actually conducted with humans. These aren't hypothetical human effects; they are actual effects of fasting, measured by scientists in a lab. I look forward to more of this type of research.

Besides this specific research study, scientists all over the world are reporting findings related to fasting and longevity. Here is just a small sampling of some recent findings:

- As we get older, the mitochondria of our cells lose the ability to process energy efficiently, which leads to both aging and age-related diseases. Our cells also lose the ability to dispose of "junk proteins," and this can lead to the accumulation of excess proteins that lead to the development of diseases such as ALS (amyotrophic lateral sclerosis) and Alzheimer's. In 2017, researchers from Harvard University reported that both exercise and fasting (even for brief periods) enhance the cells' ability to dispose of some of these "junky" proteins that cause diseases by enhancing the function of our mitochondrial networks.[7] This should lead to a reduced likelihood of developing age-related diseases, which could then increase life span. One of the scientists involved in this research referred to it as turning on the "cellular vacuum cleaner," and I love to think of my body vacuuming out the junk during my daily fast!

- We know that as we age, we become more susceptible to maladies like cardiovascular disease. Vascular aging plays a significant role in this process, as the vessels become sensitive and more subject to damage over time. In 2018, researchers at Georgia State University identified a molecule with antiaging effects on the vascular system.[8] They found that one of the molecules the body produces during fasting (beta-hydroxybutyrate, or BHB) promotes cell division and prevents cellular aging within the blood vessels and lymphatic vessels of our vascular systems. They believe this may help us keep our blood vessels "young" and healthy. I love the sound of that!

- As we age, our intestinal stem cells lose their regenerative abilities, and it takes longer for the intestines to recover from infection or injury. Biologists at MIT found that a twenty-four-hour fast can reverse age-related loss of intestinal stem cell function.[9] In this 2018 study, they found evidence that "fasting induces a metabolic switch in the intestinal stem cells, from utilizing carbohydrates to burning fat." As a result of the metabolic changes, they saw enhanced function and cellular regeneration. While we can't see inside our intestinal tracts, I love the idea that the lining of my intestines is youthful and strong.

- In 2018, researchers performed a comprehensive review of the scientific literature on fasting.[10] This type of research summary is important, because scientists examine all the previous research they can find and put it together into a comprehensive big picture of what the research is showing us as a whole. In their paper, they examined both time-restricted eating (the eating-window approach) and various alternate-daily fasting strategies (the up-and-down-day approach). (More about what these IF terms mean in later chapters!) In their analysis, they described how fasting allows our bodies to shift from burning glucose for energy to obtaining energy from fatty acids and their by-products, ketones. When the body flips this metabolic switch, it can access fat stores while preserving lean muscle mass (sound familiar?). Also, based on their analysis of the scientific literature on fasting, the researchers report that fasting "may optimize physiological functioning, enhance performance, and slow the aging and disease processes." We are definitely not surprised, are we?

- In 2018, scientists at the National Institute on Aging put mice on two distinct diets (meaning they fed each diet group a carefully developed mouse diet), and within each of these diet groups, they divided the mice into subgroups based on different eating patterns.[11] One subgroup could eat around the clock, another received the same type of food but only 70 percent of the amount (leading to a 30 percent restriction in calories), and the third group received one meal with the same number of calories enjoyed by the mouse group that was fed around the clock. The researchers found that "health and longevity improved with increased fasting time, regardless of what the mice ate or how many calories they consumed." That is very cool, because the difference wasn't from the foods themselves or from the restriction in calories; the difference was attributable to the longer period of fasting. The mice that ate one meal a day, which was the longest fasting period examined, "seemed to have a longer lifespan and better outcomes for common age-related liver disease and metabolic disorders." Yes, these were mice, but the researchers are hoping to expand the research to other animals and then eventually to humans.

I could literally go on and on and on, but I will stop myself because hopefully this small sampling is enough to convince you that the research into fasting and longevity is both exciting and promising.

In these first three chapters, I have shown you *why* we choose intermittent fasting as a lifestyle:

- IF ignites our fat-burning superpower!

- IF is the health plan with a side effect of weight loss!

- IF is the real-life fountain of youth!

Now that you understand the *why,* I imagine that you are ready for me to teach you the *how*: how to develop your own personalized intermittent fasting program that will help you achieve some of the exciting health benefits of IF and maybe some of that magical fat-burning superpower from chapter 1 as well. (Who am I kidding? Most of us start IF for the weight loss, and then we stick around for the health benefits, so let's definitely design a program that helps you do both! Win-win, baby!) Keep reading to learn everything you need to know to become an intermittent faster!

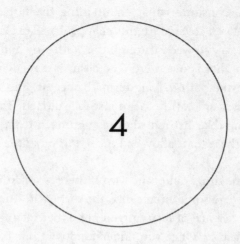

4

THE MAGIC IS IN THE CLEAN FAST! LEARN *WHY* WE FAST CLEAN

Before you start fasting, you need to understand how to ensure you are getting all the health and fat-burning benefits from fasting. The key to this lies in understanding the magic of the clean fast! This chapter will teach you the *why* behind the clean-fast recommendations, and the next chapter will teach you the *how*. So, read both! But if you're anxious to get started, you have my permission to flip right to the next chapter and read that first, as long as you promise me you will come back to this one to understand the reasons behind the recommendations. I find that I am more likely to follow a recommendation when I fully understand why it is important, so don't neglect this important step in the learning process.

These two chapters are the most important in the whole book, because there are so many misconceptions floating around about what's safe to consume while maintaining the fasted state. Don't worry! I've got you covered. In this chapter, I will explain everything you need to know to wade through the confusing and often contradictory advice that is out there. The clean fast really is a nonnegotiable step on the path to long-term IF success, and I want you to experience the magic of the clean fast for yourself. The clean fast is also something that distinguishes my approach from the multitude of others out there that "allow" a *little of this* or a *little of that* during the fast.

Let's get one thing out of the way. If there is something called the *clean fast,* is there something called the *dirty fast*? The answer is no. Based on the science of fasting, you are either fasting clean or you aren't really fasting. Once you understand why this is true, you will understand that a dirty fast doesn't really exist.

Where did the term *clean fast* come from? It actually was born in my IF support group in 2017, after my first book, *Delay, Don't Deny,* had been released. One day, I said "fasting clean" to describe the most effective way to fast, and the term stuck. Before I knew it, it was part of our support group's lingo. And over the past year or so, I have seen the phrase begin popping up in other fasting communities as well. I am thrilled to have brought the term *clean fast* to the world, because I think it describes what we want out of the fasting period: it is the time where our bodies can "clean" and repair (thanks, autophagy!), so keeping the fast itself clean will ensure that our bodies can do all the behind-the-scenes "cleaning" we want to experience during the fast. Once you understand the purpose of the clean fast, you will want to protect that sacred part of the day at all costs.

Never forget that the period of the day when you are fasting is designed to be a rest from food. This is a key to understanding the principles of the clean fast: avoid anything that *is* food for your body or that makes your body *think* food is on the way.

To fully understand and embrace the recommendations for the clean fast, we have to be clear on *why* we are fasting. During the clean fast, these are our main goals:

1. Keep insulin levels as low as possible during the fast.

2. Tap into our own fat stores for fuel.

3. Experience increased autophagy and all the upcycling that comes along with it.

Once we understand the goals of the clean fast, we can easily understand how to make those things happen:

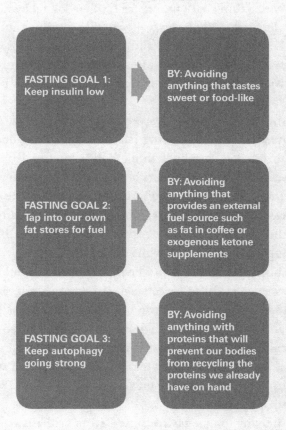

FASTING GOAL 1: Keep insulin low

BY: Avoiding anything that tastes sweet or food-like

FASTING GOAL 2: Tap into our own fat stores for fuel

BY: Avoiding anything that provides an external fuel source such as fat in coffee or exogenous ketone supplements

FASTING GOAL 3: Keep autophagy going strong

BY: Avoiding anything with proteins that will prevent our bodies from recycling the proteins we already have on hand

Let's unpack each of these three goals one by one and learn how to specifically apply each to the clean fast. When we are done, you'll be equipped with the knowledge to keep your fast squeaky clean!

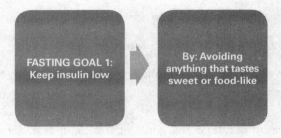

I want you to think back to chapter 1, where I taught you about insulin and what it does in the body. Recall that insulin is antilipolytic, meaning it is anti–fat burning, and therefore high levels of insulin keep us from accessing our fat stores effectively. For that reason, we want to *avoid* ingesting anything during the fast that would make our bodies secrete more insulin.

What makes your body release insulin? Eating food, of course, and we already know that eating isn't fasting. But so does tasting anything that makes your body think food is coming.

Sweetness and food-like flavors both send the signal to your brain that food is on the way and insulin is needed *pronto*! The very taste of sweetness or food-like flavors, even if you don't actually swallow anything, initiates the *cephalic phase insulin release,* or CPIR, which is something we want to avoid while fasting.

I remember back to the days when I was obese. I would start the day with sweetened coffee (sweetened with zero-calorie stevia!), sip on a diet soda (I always had one on my desk during the school day!), enjoy tantalizing herbal teas with dessert-like names (oh so delicious, and zero calories!), and chew sugar-free gum (sweetened with Xylitol, because it was "good for my teeth"!). Basically, I had something sweetened and/or flavored going into my mouth *All. Day. Long.* Like a toddler with a sippy cup.

Every time my tongue tasted those flavors or that sweetness, my brain got the message that I needed a burst of insulin to manage the calories that were on the way . . . except that the calories never came, because I was using zero-calorie sweeteners and products with added flavors. Unfortunately, our brains don't know the difference between regular sweeteners (like honey or sugar) and zero-calorie/artificial sweeteners (such as stevia, aspartame, or sucralose) or flavors from actual food (such as strawberries or chocolate) and zero-calorie-added flavors (including both natural and artificial food-like flavors).

Do you remember the saying, "You can't fool Mother Nature"? Well, these artificial sweeteners and added flavors actually *are* fooling Mother Nature, and it has definite consequences for our bodies. Our brains don't understand that we have figured out how to make something that tastes like food but actually isn't food, so they prepare for the calories . . . that never come.

How does this work? Our taste buds send signals to our brains to prepare our bodies to process the food that is incoming. As an example, sweet, sour, and umami foods increase saliva secretion (which helps our bodies prepare for digestion and food absorption) while bitter flavors (such as black coffee and plain tea) do not have this effect.[1] Sweet and food-like flavors are linked to more than just a saliva release, though, because the body expects carbohydrates. Besides increasing saliva production, the body also releases insulin as soon as sweetness is detected so that the required amount of insulin will be available as soon as the body needs it. This is the cephalic phase insulin response (CPIR) I mentioned earlier.[2]

Let's learn the science of how the CPIR works. Within two minutes of tasting sweetness, the body releases insulin. The amount of insulin peaks at four minutes and returns to baseline levels within eight to ten minutes. (This is why it's okay to brush your teeth during the fast, by the way: even though your toothpaste may have a hint of sweetness, insulin goes back down pretty quickly after such a brief encounter.) But this also explains why it is *not* okay to drink a sweetened beverage or chew sweetened gum. You don't just have one sip or one chew and go about your day. No, you drink that sweetened cup of coffee or diet soda over a long period, and each time you sip, your body continues to release insulin in response. I think back to the way I lived prior to understanding the clean fast. I was constantly nursing a sweetened coffee or a flavored water or a diet soda. I was pretty much CPIRing myself during all waking hours. (*CPIRing* is not an official scientific term, and I just made it up, but I'm sure you understand what I meant.)

There are numerous studies that illustrate the relationship between tasting sweetness or food-like flavors and CPIR (insulin release). The one that convinced me was a 2008 human study that showed a "significant increase of plasma insulin concentration" when participants swished a sweetened solution around in their mouths (in this study, they tested both sucrose and saccharin).[3] The subjects didn't even swallow! All they did was swish and spit.

There have been other convincing studies. In a 2017 study, scientists found that subjects who were overweight had a "significant" CPIR in response to the taste of sucralose.[4] And in a study from 1993, scientists examined the difference in insulin response between subjects of normal weight and those who were obese. They found that the obese subjects with elevated fasting insulin levels (meaning that they *started* with higher baseline insulin levels!) had an *even greater* CPIR than the normal-weight subjects.[5] Why is this important? Well, if you have been overweight (or obese) for a while, and if you have higher levels of insulin at all times, you may release even *more* insulin in response to a sweet taste than your skinny friend. That just doesn't seem fair, does it?

Here's one more study that may be even more convincing for any skeptics out there. In a 2007 rat study, scientists measured their insulin response to sweet tastes. As we'd expect, the rats had an insulin release after consuming sweetened water (they tested both sucrose and saccharin). But this is where it gets interesting! In the second part of the experiment, the scientists cut the nerves from the tongue so their brains could no longer get the message of sweetness. Voilà! No more CPIR. The *taste* was what mattered.[6]

Even in the face of the evidence I just shared, it may surprise you to know that the "sweet taste and insulin release" debate remains one of the biggest sticking points for many people, and there are those out there who ridicule the concept completely. (Of course, most of those people are also stuck in the "it's all about the calories" mindset, which is why they can't quite believe that something with zero calories could prevent your body from burning fat. It can be hard to unlearn something you've always taken as gospel.)

Why is this controversial? Well, as with many topics in the health field, you can find studies (and resulting conclusions) that contradict one another. That's right! You can find studies like the ones I shared that show there is an insulin response to sweet tastes, and you can also find studies that show there is *not* an insulin response to sweet tastes! As a result, some people claim that one sweetener may be connected to insulin release while another is somehow magically exempt. (Ask yourself this question: How would the body know the difference between one artificial sweetener and another? On the tongue, sweet is sweet!)

So, what do we do when faced with contradictory information? What if you watch an internet video or read a blog post that sounds very scientific and claims that sweetener XYZ is perfectly fine while fasting? For me, it's an easy decision. I personally want to err on the side of caution. If there is a possibility that something is going to cause me to release insulin during the fast, I am going to avoid it. *Nothing* gets between me and my fat-burning superpower!

Trust me when I tell you that *no one* wanted to have stevia during the fast more than I did. Once I learned the science behind insulin release, I searched and searched for a rationale that would allow me to keep stevia in my coffee (and allow me to continue chewing gum, drinking zero-calorie sodas, sipping flavored waters, enjoying my fruity and sweet herbal teas, etc.). Once I became truly honest with myself, however, I realized there wasn't one.

When I decided to eliminate those sweet and food-like flavors during the fast, it changed the way I experienced intermittent fasting and made the process truly effortless. And there is one more thing I want to emphasize: prior to implementing a truly clean fast, I had also started to experience a slow but steady weight regain, and the minute I gave up stevia and other sweet tastes during the fast, that weight gain completely reversed and I went on to lose two more jeans sizes over the next year, even though I had declared myself at my goal weight over a year earlier. Yep. Eliminating the sweetness during the fast made a huge difference for my body.

Now that we understand the relationship between sweet tastes and insulin release, let's move on to the second fasting goal:

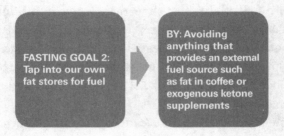

This is a tough one for many people because there is a lot of chatter in the intermittent fasting world that insists that consuming fat is "just fine" during the fast because it won't lead to insulin release. Bring on the butter in your coffee! Chug some MCT oil! Get yourself "into ketosis faster" by drinking a magical ketone drink! (No, no, and no, y'all.)

There is a mistaken thought that consuming excess fat or exogenous ketones during the fast will somehow magically make your body burn *more* of your own fat than if you fasted clean. Let's examine the science behind both energy sources and understand why we don't want to include them in our fast.

First, remember that one of the goals of intermittent fasting is to tap into our own fat stores for fuel during the fast. So, it makes sense that you would want to skip any added fats and oils! As an example, there's a popular coffee drink that includes ingredients like butter, coconut oil, and/or MCT oil. Many people find it to be absolutely delicious, and there are claims that it will boost both your fat-burning potential and give you amazing energy. (Well, it does give you energy—the energy from all that fat you just consumed!) Do you know what else gives you great energy? Fasting clean! When your body becomes metabolically flexible, you make ketones from your stored fat. BOOM! You'll feel energetic and mentally sharp.

Here's one more thing to keep in mind. While I'm going to teach you in chapter 15 that all calories aren't treated the same in the body (so I don't recommend counting calories in general), does it make sense that consuming hundreds of calories of excess fat in your coffee would be a good fat-loss strategy? Think about this. Fat you consume gives you energy that you need to use *before* tapping into your own fat stores! I know I would prefer to burn my own excess fat from my thighs rather than the fat from my coffee cup.

Now, let's talk about taking exogenous ketones during the fast. You probably have a friend who wants to sell you this magical potion to "*get you into ketosis!*" and "*boost fat burning!*" They sound too good to be true, just as all miracle supplements that come along.

What exactly are exogenous ketones? Ketones are energy, so when you take in a ketone supplement, you are literally taking in a source of fuel for your body. Here is something that is important to understand: our goal isn't *having* ketones in our bodies; the goal is *making* ketones from our own body fat, just as nature intended, for *free*. Yes, taking exogenous ketones will give you a positive on a ketone test, because you literally just ingested those ketones—you didn't produce them. You swallowed them!

While the people who want to sell you exogenous ketones will tell you that their ketones will somehow make your body burn your own fat "better" and somewhat magically, akin to rainbows and unicorns, think about it from your body's perspective. If you have a source of ketones coming in from a supplement, why on earth would you need to make any from your own fat? Instead of using a supplement, tap into *your* fat-burning superpower! For FREE! Of course, if you have a neurological condition like epilepsy or Alzheimer's that can benefit from extra ketones, then taking exogenous ketones therapeutically may be a fantastic option for you. If your goal is burning your own fat for fuel, however, it's a "nope" from me.

So now that we understand why we don't want to take in any added fuel sources during the fast, let's look at fasting goal 3:

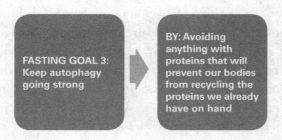

If you think back to what you learned about autophagy from the previous chapters, I'm sure that you don't want to do anything that will prevent your body from ramping up these processes during the fast!

What halts autophagy? Eating, of course, but we specifically want to avoid taking in any types of proteins during the fast. This includes collagen supplements and bone broth, as well as the supplements that are sold to us as pre- or post-workout products. As an example of why this matters, in a 2010 study, scientists found that supplementation with leucine (an amino acid) decreased autophagy markers in the study's participants.[7] In addition to this effect, the protein also led to an increase in the participants' insulin levels. That's a double whammy!

So, when fasting, we want our bodies to break down our old junky proteins and reuse them. For that reason, avoid taking in a new source of protein.

Now that we have explored all three of the fasting goals and the science behind each of them, you should understand why the clean fast is so important. It's time to make sure you are fully equipped to apply this information to your fasting practice!

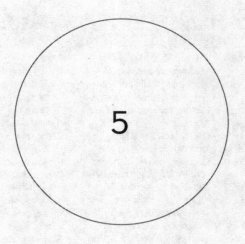

5

KEEP IT CLEAN!
LEARN *HOW* WE FAST CLEAN

Now that you fully understand the goals of the clean fast, it's important to know how to apply this to your life. That's what this chapter is for! When you're done reading, you'll have the tools to figure out how to keep your fast squeaky clean.

As you know, I am a retired teacher, so I have included something in this chapter for everyone in our clean-fast classroom!

Perhaps you are a rule follower. (Teacher's pet? No problem! You keep our classrooms running smoothly.) If so, here is a handy-dandy graphic that you can use to figure out what you can and can't have during the fast, and I know you will appreciate having it all laid out for you in easy black and white.

WHAT IS A "CLEAN FAST"?		
YES!	**MAYBE . . .**	**NO!**
• Water (unflavored) • Black coffee (unflavored) • Any plain tea brewed from actual dried leaves only (black tea, green tea, etc., unflavored varieties only, loose or in tea bags) • Mineral water, club soda, sparkling water, or seltzer water (unflavored) • Minerals/electrolytes/salt (with no additives or flavors) • Medications as prescribed by your health care provider	We call this the "gray area": • Peppermint essential oil for breath freshening only, NOT for water-enhancing (*select food-grade and use sparingly*) • Herbal tea with a bitter flavor profile • Vitamins and supplements (*There is no easy answer for all vitamins and supplements. Any that are clearly food-like or listed in the "No" column should be taken within your eating window.*)	• Food • Flavored water • Flavored coffee • Fruity, sweet, or matcha teas • Diet sodas • Natural or artificial sweeteners • Gum or mints • Food-like flavors of any type (*fruit juices, fruit flavors, etc.*) • Bone broth, broth, or bouillon • Fat, including coconut oil, MCT oil, butter, etc. • Cream, creamers, milk, or milk substitutes (*of any amount or type*) • Supplements such as collagen, pre-workouts, BCAAs, exogenous ketones, etc.

When living an intermittent fasting lifestyle, the real magic happens during the clean fast! Whenever you aren't sure if something is okay for the clean fast, look at the ingredients and compare them against this chart. If it has only ingredients from the Yes column, it's fine. If it has ingredients from the No column, you know it doesn't work. And if it is something in the gray area, it may or may not work for you.

IMPORTANT: Don't experiment with anything from the gray area until after you complete the twenty-eight-day FAST Start. At that point, you should know how your body feels during the clean fast. If you then experiment with a gray area item and you find it makes you hungry or shaky or nauseous within about an hour (or sooner), that is a clear signal that it doesn't work well for you during the fast. When something makes you ravenous or shaky, that is a sign that your body released insulin and insulin did its job and therefore lowered your blood glucose (leading to the shakiness or hunger). If the item is okay for you, you probably won't notice any difference in hunger or energy levels; you'll feel the same as you did when fasting clean. If that happens, congratulations! That item is probably fine for you. By the way, this is *never* an excuse for trying anything from the No list. The "does it make me hungry or shaky" test isn't foolproof, and remember that you don't want to risk breaking your fast. Everything on the No list is *always* a no.

Perhaps you aren't a teacher's pet but find yourself to be more of a "*But WHY?*" person. If so, I have a section for you, as well. I am going to go through all the items one by one and explain why each is either a great choice for the fast or a not-so-great choice. After reading this, you will never have to ask if something is going to work during the clean fast; you will be equipped to use this information to figure it out for yourself.

THE YES COLUMN: WHY?	
Water (*unflavored*)	Water is a great choice during a fast! While you don't want to overdo it, drink whenever you are thirsty. Make sure that you are not adding any flavor enhancers or fruit/food slices to your water. Keep it "water flavored" only. Here's a tip: Consider making yourself a mug of hot water during the fast. Maybe that sounds crazy (or even sad), but it is one of my favorite beverages when the weather is cooler. A nice mug of hot water hits the spot, and it is surprisingly soothing! We call it Em tea (say that quickly to get the joke).

Black coffee (*unflavored*)	Why is coffee okay for fasting, when most of the other clean-fast recommendations have to do with avoiding flavor? Isn't coffee a "flavor"? Yes, but black coffee has a bitter flavor profile, and the body shouldn't release insulin in response to a bitter flavor.[1] You do want to avoid any naturally or artificially flavored coffee beans and stick to the unflavored varieties.
	     Coffee has many benefits that make it perfect for the clean fast. First, coffee is linked to increased autophagy![2] I remind myself of that fact as I enjoy my daily espresso. Coffee also stimulates fat burning and may help us deplete our liver glycogen stores more quickly, which would get us into the fasted state sooner (though it spares glycogen in the muscles, which helps us work out in the fasted state).[3,4]
	     Now for the elephant in the room, and the *number one* problem new IFers face:
	     "Gin, I can't drink my coffee black. I can't. Don't make me do this."

cont.

Let's imagine that you aren't a black coffee drinker and you actually are more accustomed to drinking your coffee in a form I refer to as a "hot milkshake." What can you add to coffee to make it more delicious? NOTHING, and I am not kidding. Check the No list. Pretty much everything you could think of adding to coffee is listed in the No column.

You may think there is no way you would ever be able to adjust to drinking your coffee black, but you absolutely can. Hold your nose, drink it down, and give your taste buds a couple of weeks to adjust to the bitterness. You'll find that you absolutely can acquire a taste for black coffee! There are a couple of strategies that some have found to help the coffee adjustment phase: add a tiny pinch of salt to cut the bitterness or dilute your coffee with hot water to make it weaker.

Here's something else that is cool about acquiring a taste for black coffee. Many of us in the intermittent fasting community have found that the bitterness of black coffee has opened up our palates in a miraculous way. That's certainly been true for me. After adjusting to the taste of black coffee, I suddenly became able to tolerate *other* bitter flavors, as well. This opened up a world of vegetables to me. Suddenly, I enjoyed bitter vegetables, whereas before I couldn't stand the taste. I totally credit this change to my acquired taste for black coffee. Since I am not alone in experiencing this phenomenon, see if it happens for you! It's one more reason to embrace black coffee rather than tell yourself that you can't. #IfGinCanYOUCan

And if you *really don't* want to drink black coffee?

Don't drink coffee at all! That's okay, too. Coffee itself is not a requirement.

Any plain tea brewed from actual dried tea leaves only (*black tea, green tea, etc., unflavored varieties only, loose or in tea bags*)	As I've already said, bitter flavors are fine during the fast, and plain tea fits that description. Check the ingredients and choose a variety where the *only* ingredient is tea. Any Yes column tea comes from the *Camellia sinensis* plant, and varieties include black tea, green tea, white tea, oolong tea, and pu-erh tea. (In this context, "white tea" refers to a variety made from minimally processed tea leaves, and *not* milky tea, which some countries call "white tea.") Why is tea such a great choice? Tea has numerous health benefits, and compounds found within tea (and specifically in green tea) are linked to increased autophagy.[5]
Mineral water, club soda, sparkling water, or seltzer water (*unflavored*)	Sparkling mineral or soda waters are an excellent choice during the fast. Make sure to avoid any with added flavors or sweeteners. *Tonic water is not part of a clean fast, as tonic water has added sweeteners.*

Minerals/electrolytes/salt (*with no additives or flavors*)	Minerals/electrolytes/salt do not break the fast. It is important to realize that when fasting, you may be more prone to an electrolyte imbalance, particularly if you are drinking a great deal of water.[6] You can add minerals or an electrolyte supplement to your water to help prevent that from happening. Make sure to check the ingredients list and choose something that doesn't contain any ingredients from the No list. Unflavored mineral drops are a great choice. Avoid options with citric acid, which can add a tangy flavor. Safety note: Drinking *too much* water while fasting could actually be dangerous. This happens when excessive water intake "flushes out" the concentration of electrolytes in your body. Symptoms include a headache or mental confusion. If you are fasting and you've been drinking water excessively, pay attention to those danger signs and seek medical care immediately if you suspect you've had too much water.
Medications as prescribed by your health care provider	When you need medications, you take them. Period. That being said, never hesitate to have a conversation with your doctor or pharmacist about your specific prescriptions. It's possible that you may need to have dosages or timings adjusted. Some may need to be taken on an empty stomach, while others may need to be taken with food. Fasting may also affect dosages. Work with your health care provider to develop a plan that works with your body, your health conditions, and your goals.

THE NO COLUMN: WHY?	
Food	Please don't ask if you can eat something during the fast. You cannot. Eating is never fasting. If something is food, it's not part of a clean fast. Even if it's bitter. Even if it's tiny. Even if you watched an internet video that said it was okay. Repeat after me: if something is food, it isn't part of fasting.
Flavored water	Fasting goal number one is to avoid anything that may stimulate CPIR (insulin release), so avoid adding any flavors to your water. Yes, this includes *anything* that you can think of (other than perhaps a sprinkle of salt). If something adds flavor to your water, don't add it. "But, Gin, what about . . ." NO. "*How about . . .*" STILL NO. Embrace water that tastes like . . . water.

cont.

Flavored coffee	There are many flavors of coffee out there: Hazelnut. *Yum!* French Vanilla. *Absolutely delicious!* Caramel Extravaganza. *Sounds delightful!* And that is exactly what your brain will think when you drink them. Sorry, y'all. Avoid flavored coffees during the fast. You don't want your brain to think you are having a delicious dessert. Stick to plain and bitter black coffee only.
Fruity, sweet, or matcha teas	As you already have learned, a sweet or food-like flavor will stimulate CPIR. So, avoid all these types of tea during the fast and save them for your eating window. What about matcha? Matcha is made from a powder that you mix with water. Rather than brewing the tea leaves and discarding them, you actually consume them. Is that enough to break the fast? I wouldn't risk it. Yes, there is a quantity of matcha powder that would definitely break the fast, and I can't tell you with any certainty what that threshold would be. So, follow the rule of thumb: when in doubt, leave it out.
Diet sodas	You shouldn't need me to tell you this if you read the last chapter: sweet taste = insulin release. So, you absolutely don't want to consume any diet sodas during the fast.
Natural or artificial flavors	Our goal is to avoid anything with food-like flavors during the fast, so avoid any products that have either natural or artificial flavors on the ingredients list. Here's something else that makes natural or artificial flavors so problematic. Food manufacturers hide all sorts of things in foods using the words *natural flavors* or *artificial flavors*. You literally have no idea what they might include or how it might break the fast. Save the flavors for your eating window, when you can have any flavor you want.
Natural or artificial sweeteners	Again, remember that sweet taste = insulin release. No matter what *NEW! Amazing new sweetener! Safe for fasting!* they may try to come up with (and the more mainstream fasting becomes, the more they will try), if it is sweet, you don't want to include it as part of a clean fast. One thing that confuses many people: sweeteners are often marketed as "*no glycemic response!*" and that makes people think they don't affect the fast. "Glycemic response" means that it raises blood sugar. Remember: we are trying to avoid insulin release, and that is not the same thing.
Gum or mints	This fits into the sweet taste = insulin release category. There are no commercially produced gums or mints that fit into the "safe for clean fasting" category because all of them contain sweeteners and flavors.

Food-like flavors of any type (*fruit juices, fruit flavors, etc.*)	As I have already told you, food-like flavors trick your brain into thinking that food is on the way.
	
	    This includes things like lemon wedges, cucumber slices, apple cider vinegar, pickle juice, mint leaves, herbs, even citric acid, which adds a tangy flavor. The possibilities are endless, and I named only a few.
	
	    Bottom line: if something has the flavor of any food, avoid it during the fast.

Bone broth, broth, or bouillon	Broth and bouillon are often thought of as a great "diet food" because they are low in calories. You know what else, though? They taste like food. Avoid all things that taste like food. Bone broth is a particularly tricky one because there are things called *bone broth fasts* that sound very healthy. Well, bone broth is full of protein. If you remember fasting goal number three, we want to avoid anything with protein. Save the bone broth (or any broth) for your eating window.
Fats, including coconut oil, MCT oil, butter, etc.	Recall fasting goal number two, which is to tap into our fat stores for fuel. For that reason, avoid any added fats during the fast. Consuming fats absolutely *will* keep you from burning your *own* stored fat.

Cream, creamers, milk, or milk substitutes (*of any amount or type*)	Let's think about this one. What exactly is milk? It's nature's perfect food designed for mammal babies to eat during the time when they are growing at the greatest rate of their lives.
	
	    Does that sound like fasting? No, it sounds like food.
	
	    There is no type of cream, creamer, or milk that you can have during the fast. It doesn't matter if it is milk from an animal source or "milk" from a plant source. Avoid anything that is a milk or milk substitute.

Supplements, such as collagen, pre-workouts, BCAAs, exogenous ketones, etc.	Recall fasting goal number three, which is to avoid protein during the fast. Most of these supplements have protein in them. Many also contain sweeteners or added flavors. Exogenous ketones are a source of fuel for the body. I promise you don't need or want any of these during the fast.

THE MAYBE COLUMN: WHY?	
Peppermint essential oil for breath freshening only, *not* for water enhancing (*select food-grade and use sparingly*)	Face it—sometimes we have bad breath, and we need to do something when we have to get up close and personal with other people. Many people can use a tiny drop of peppermint essential oil for breath freshening during the fast with no issues.

cont.

	Why not use it as a water enhancer? Remember that we aren't trying to make fasting into a flavor adventure. A tiny drop for fresh breath is brief. A beverage, on the other hand, goes on and on. Important note: All essential oils are not created equal. If you are using peppermint essential oil in your mouth, select a food-grade variety, and use it both sparingly and carefully. It's best to research the safe use of essential oils before proceeding. Follow recommendations from each specific essential oil manufacturer.
Herbal tea with a bitter flavor profile	I wanted to write a whole chapter called "Why Are There So Many Beverages Called *Tea* and Why Are Most of Them Not Actually Made from the Plant Officially Known as Tea," but that seemed excessive. Based on my research, there are exactly eleventy-bazillion products you can buy that have "tea" on the label, and they may be made from a variety of leaves, herbs, or miscellaneous plant parts. Some are made from mushrooms, and others are made from roots. It is enough to make your head spin! We know that sweet or fruity flavors cause CPIR, or insulin release. Bitter flavors do not. So, whenever you are considering an herbal tea made from anything beyond *actual tea* leaves, make sure it has a bitter flavor profile. As I've already mentioned, a bitter taste is not associated with CPIR. Always avoid any teas that have food-like flavors.
Vitamins and supplements	There is no easy answer for all vitamins and supplements. Any that are clearly food-like (or are listed in the No column) should be taken in your eating window. Many vitamins and supplements are absorbed better when taken with food, though some need to be taken on an empty stomach. If your health care provider recommends that you take specific vitamins and/or supplements, discuss appropriate timings with him or her.

Hopefully, these lists have equipped you with all the information you need to decide if something fits into the clean fast. If you are still not sure if something is clean-fast approved, I like to follow this rule of thumb: when in doubt, leave it out.

Maybe, though, you aren't a teacher's pet or a "*But WHY?*" student . . . you're actually a rebel, and you still aren't convinced. (I see you there, rebel, needing just a bit more from me before you commit. I understand where you are coming from; really, I do. You rebels make us better teachers, and good teachers actually appreciate the opportunity you give us to hone our skills.)

If you are a rebel, then you may not believe me when I tell you that a little sweetener in your coffee or a wedge of lemon in your water is not part of a clean fast. You're not alone! There are a lot of rebels out there who have had to test it out for themselves.

I have some stories from experienced intermittent fasters at the end of this chapter that should help convince you that it's not just me; you can rest assured that these clean-fast suggestions have been vetted by hundreds of thousands of IFers.

If that doesn't do it, I have designed the Clean Fast Challenge just for YOU! Once you take me up on the clean-fast challenge, you, too, will be a believer. I promise.

Take the *Clean Fast Challenge*!

Before I share the personal stories with you, let's learn about the Clean Fast Challenge! First, take the time to Google "Pepsi Challenge video" and watch it. (And enjoy the fun clothes and hairdos from the early 1980s, when the Pepsi Challenge was a thing.) Go ahead. I'll wait.

If you're of my generation or older, you'll remember this ad campaign well. Pepsi was the underdog in the cola wars and wanted to prove to the world that it was superior in taste to the more popular Coke. The Pepsi Challenge was born! The commercials showed one surprised consumer after another choosing Pepsi in a blind taste test. From one of the ads: "More people prefer the taste of Pepsi to Coca-Cola. Take the Pepsi Challenge. Let your taste decide."

So, what in the heck does this have to do with fasting? It's simple! I want you to take my Clean Fast Challenge. If you still aren't convinced that _____ is a problem during the fast (fill in the blank with whatever you are resisting), you're a perfect candidate for this challenge.

Here's how it works. I want you to commit to six to eight weeks of fasting clean Gin-style. Absolutely no deviations from the Yes list. After the six to eight weeks (no cheating!), try whatever you are unsure about. Pay attention to how your body feels after consuming it. I am convinced that you will be a believer.

After all, "More people prefer the Clean Fast. Take the Clean Fast Challenge. Let your body decide."

Let's hear about this truth straight from the mouths of some experienced IFers!

Laurie Lewis	When I first started fasting I thought herbal tea was OK, and I drank it throughout the day. I was hungry ALL the time! Once I learned to eliminate those teas, I switched to plain water, the hunger would come in waves, but it wasn't constant. My mind was freed up to go about my day, and I wasn't so pained by gnawing, shaky, ravenous hunger.
Angie Stark	Before I discovered what constituted a "clean fast", I struggled greatly to make it to a 16 hour fast. This was the case for about my first month (started in December 2018). After reading about the clean fast, I realized that gum breaks a fast! Now, it seems so clear, but at that time, I had NO IDEA. I mean—gum!!! Anyway, once I realized that was the case, I stopped chewing gum outside of my eating window, and I have been clean fasting every day since.
Kiki W from Boston	Clean fast actually helps push me through the fasting window. I experienced shakiness while I was doing a dirty fast by accident and it made me hangry and want to binge everything after I opened my window. I can't recommend enough the importance of the clean fast.
Justin Claypool	For a long time I have been doing what I THOUGHT was intermittent fasting. I was replacing breakfast with fat/keto coffee, then eating all my solid food in a four hour window later in the day. I was constantly hungry all day after my coffee. Then I read about the clean fast and found out my fast was dirty! I started doing a true clean fast, drinking my coffee black and not having flavored water during my fasting time. Not only did I break the weight plateau I had been on forever but I was no longer hungry, my skin cleared up, and I started seeing more of the IF benefits everyone raved about!

Stephanie Riggins	Thought I was Intermittent Fasting for months but seeing absolutely no weight loss results. Turns out drinking a protein shake in the morning is NOT clean fasting. I thought since I wasn't eating solid foods, I was fasting! Ditched the protein shake and clean fasted noon-8 pm, changed NOTHING ELSE, ate what I wanted to in my eating window, denied and deprived myself of absolutely nothing, and I'm down almost 50 pounds in 7 months. There is magic in a squeaky clean fast!
Noreen Barrese	I did this backwards. As a new faster, right from the start, I clean fasted. Day 1 I started with clean fast and was amazed how long I could fast without feeling shaky or hangry. After 82 days of squeaky clean fasts I purposely added my favorite cream to my favorite flavored coffee. The first thing I noticed was that it wasn't nearly as yummy as I had recalled. Halfway through the cup, I was ravenously hungry, starting to shake and felt weak. I needed food and needed it now! I typically break my fasts with nuts, fruit, cheese and build normal hunger. Dirty fasting or breaking with sugary coffee is something I will never do again.
Carrie	When I first started IF, I was using a popular "healthy" drink first thing in the morning because their company claimed that it was not breaking my fast. Funny enough I wasn't losing weight. After a few weeks when I realized that I was in fact breaking my fast, I decided to ditch the drink. Not only did I start losing weight and fasting became easier, I started saving a lot of money!
Chris K from Bowling Green KY	Approx. 7 months into my new L*IF*E's journey I found I had stopped seeing weight loss and, even more discouraging, NSVs. I started to see some pounds creep back and I was starting to get hangry before my windows—yikes! Back to IF 'boot camp' for me! I reread Gin's "Delay, Don't Deny" as if I were rediscovering IF for the first time. The light bulb lit up! I was trying cut down a tree with a dull saw!! I'd never cut out artificial sweeteners or heavy cream in my coffee, before my open windows; in essence shortening my fasts considerably. Since embracing the 'clean fast' the hangryness is gone, NSVs are back, and slow and steady weight loss returned. I've never felt better.
Kim from Louisiana	I tried to dirty fast at first. I was so hungry, watching the clock until I could finally break my fast. Once I started a clean fast, I noticed that fasting was so much easier. I was able to meet my goals easily and even stretch a little further. It made fasting so much easier!
Sarah from Stanmore UK	I just couldn't figure out why I could so easily fast 24, 48, even up to 72 hours without feeling hungry, but yet on occasions I would struggle and feel very hungry after just half a day. Then it hit me: mints, the days when I thought I would just have a mint so I didn't have bad breath were the days when fasting was hard. So for me the importance of the clean fast was to make it so much easier for myself. One mint spiked insulin, and it was just hard to not feel hungry. Clean fast, easy, could fast happily for a day or so.

cont.

Kristie H from Clarkston	I have never been a stranger to skipping a meal, but clean fasting is the key to making this lifestyle work long term. Once in a great while I will "mess up" and accidentally drink something that isn't part of the clean fast and within 10 minutes I'm so hungry. #gamechanger
Kim T from Illinois	As a sugar addict, specifically chocolate, when I clean fast I do not experience cravings for sweets like I have in the past. My prior attempts at healthy eating always became sabotaged by sweets. With this way of eating, I clean fast and get to eat a little sweet treat if I feel like it but I am steering the boat now. When I have fasted dirty, (prior to learning about clean fasting), I was drawn to chocolate like a moth to a flame and had absolutely no self-control.
Melinda Roman	When I added cream/artificial sweeteners to my coffee I had to work very hard to fast past lunch. I would run all over town, get a pedicure, shop and find countless ways to busy myself so I wouldn't cave to the hunger. Once I stopped adding the goodies I was able to go about my day normally without the thought of food even entering my mind. Now I'm not busy trying to distract myself from food but I'm busy with life and I have to remind myself that food is necessary! Now I'm in control. BIG difference!!
Rachel Lee	Before clean fasting I was literally counting down the hours until I could eat again. The growling emptiness kept screaming at me. I thought that by drinking sugar free drinks I would convince my digestive system it was getting something and that would appease it, yet in reality I was making it worse. Every fast was the same—I was forever keeping note of how long I had to endure until I could finally eat again. Since I discovered the clean fast I am able to forget I'm even fasting. Lunchtime comes and goes before I realize it. I'm able to get on with my life without having my attention constantly being diverted towards my empty stomach. Sure, I get hungry, but it's no longer so all encompassing and it generally passes after a short while.
Syd Crouch	When I first started fasting I still had my coffee with creamer and sweetener because so many intermittent fasting groups say that it's alright. I couldn't figure out why I wasn't getting some of the same results of autophagy, energy, and getting rid of those last 5 lbs. Then I found Gin and started clean fasting. Night and day difference. My c-section scar all but disappeared, I lost the nagging hunger during my fast, and I lost those last 5 lbs. A clean fast is what makes the fast!
Leslie from Little Rock	I wasn't going to do IF without doing it right . . . but there were times when I would have, say, cream in my coffee. First, it wasn't as great as I thought it would be and I was more hungry sooner than before. Black coffee is worth it! Unflavored water is worth it! I was so persuaded by what my co-workers were doing that I would lose my focus! Get your mind right each day and it will make you stronger to resist temptation from what others are doing and what they may expect from you!

Natalie du Toit	I started fasting on September 19, 2019, to lose weight and heal my fatigue. I had read about clean fasting but couldn't stomach unsweetened black coffee so I used stevia to help take the bitterness away. After two weeks of (dirty) fasting, I didn't notice any health benefits so I read about the importance of keeping fasts clean. I switched to a clean fast the very next day. Some health benefits I have noticed thus far are some weight loss (I weighed regularly in the beginning but after my clothes became looser without loss on the scale, I stopped weighing), a skin tag that I had had for months fell off (I'm currently monitoring another one!) and a mole on my face that has been dark brown for as long as I can remember, has become so light that I can hardly tell it's there! I have also noticed a difference with my energy levels which are getting better and better by the week.
Lynn	The first couple of months on my journey I was very careful to only drink black coffee, green tea and water. After about a year of fasting I started a job. I bought an unsweetened bottled green tea to take to work with me. I found it hard to fast during the day at work. It turned out to be the Ascorbic acid (Vitamin C) added to the bottle of green tea. Once I made my own tea minus ascorbic acid fasting went back to being easy.
Diani Maldonado	A clean fast makes all the difference; it makes it easier. The minute I decide to drink something flavorful I get hungry, even if the drink has zero calories.
R West from Vancouver, WA	I tried intermittent fasting for the first time about 6 years ago, back in the days when I thought a Paleo lifestyle was the solution to all my problems. I "fasted" but used heavy cream in my coffee and guzzled bone broth whenever I was hungry. I didn't make my own, but instead spent quite a bit of cash on grass-fed organic beef broth from a food cart in Portland, OR. I felt hungry ALL the time and gave up soon after. Clean fasting was a game changer for me! I can go for hours and hours and not even think about food! It's easy! And WAY cheaper than the dirty, expensive bone broth way!
Eddie D. Friedman	I was first exposed to fasting decades ago. I had starts and stops along the way for a variety of reasons. Three years ago, wanting to re-incorporate fasting into my life for health and weight maintenance reasons, I came across Gin's approach. I had read numerous books on fasting and considered myself knowledgeable. Aside from Gin's favorite-teacher, classroom-honed delightful, down-to-earth, user-friendly presentation, which set her apart from some authorities who had dry, overly technical styles, Gin offered a distinctively unique "rule": The Clean Fast. For years I had accepted the mostly conventional wisdom that certain substances or a limited caloric intake, for example, zero calorie but sweetened beverages, or < 50 calories of anything, were "OK" and would not disrupt the various beneficial physiological processes of fasting. So coffee with splashes of cream and stevia helped me, I erroneously believed, get through fasts.

cont.

	Gin explained how "if you're eating, you're not fasting," and urged us to adopt the Clean Fast. Now, after three years of daily clean fasting, I would never go back. Counter-intuitively, having nothing caloric or sweet tasting or hunger-triggering during our fast is actually easier, once adapted, than a small snack. Some authorities, to train compliance, "allow" for small, high fat items such as bone broth, etc., during a fast. In my experience, Gin's "Clean Fast" wins. Since learning about and following Gin's Clean Fast, my fasts are easier, more energized and create a lightness in my mood, spirit and energy that feels, well, clean. :-)
Kimberly Baltunis	I have been IF since 2012 based off another plan. I would use a pack of Stevia in my coffee and usually a diet soda each day. Some days I'd have to eat breakfast and break my fast for the day due to getting a shaky and/or nauseous feeling. A friend introduced me to Delay, Don't Deny intermittent fasting in July of 2019 and from day one using the clean fast approach I have had zero blood sugar problems, absolutely no nausea, and have never felt like I need to eat until hours into my fast when it is time to break it due to duration not an artificial sweetener. So, in a nutshell, clean fasting allows for a long fast day to day and a much better overall experience.
Gabrielle Bryen	I used to be a slave to "white" coffee, that is, with enough cream in it to make it look quite pale. I was proud, however, that my pale coffee contained no artificial sweeteners. That I saved for my espressos (because I was so "cosmopolitan"). I couldn't even fathom drinking coffee black. I lost and regained the same five pounds and I was desperate. I was tired of my clothes not fitting, of joint pain, of a protruding belly and feeling just plain old. I stumbled upon Gin and her benefits of clean fasting. Going cold turkey on the coffee was my biggest challenge. But I did it. The same old 5 lbs. quickly snowballed into 10, 20 up until a 45 lb. weight loss. In 6 months! I was shocked. I had no idea I was spiking my insulin. No wonder I couldn't lose weight! Now I can easily keep up with my 6- and 9-year-old twins and as a Mom who is older (I'm 50), I'm no longer mistaken for Grandma. I'm a clean fast ambassador!
Michelle Chlan	Before I started fasting clean, 18/6 and 16/8 were regular days for me, which was great! After I understood that stopping flavored carbonated water and fatty-coffee changed the way I was fasting, though, it became a breeze to go 20/4, and even longer with a shorter window, then eventually ADF. Had I not realized the difference in type of fasting though, I would not have been able to breeze into longer fasts. The scale had only moved around 6-8 lbs. but the body recomposition is significant, and that's what matters most.
Mary Pat	The clean fast made all of the difference in both optimizing my health (initial goal) and in achieving weight loss (pleasant and somewhat unexpected side effect).

Carrie Hague	The clean fast is truly the key to IF. I committed to the clean fast from day 1 although it took me several weeks to fully understand the importance of it. I was drinking bottled black coffee during my first 2 weeks and thought it was on the approved list. I followed the rules . . . it wasn't flavored and I added nothing to it. I was noticing that I was starving within 30 minutes of drinking it. Turns out it had citric acid as an ingredient. I immediately switched after reading tons of labels. And I've never felt that way again. I'm down 14.2 lbs in 7 weeks.
J. Holtz	I believed coffee, tea and water was a clean fast, and had the understanding that some experts allowed 50 calories of cream or bone broth if needed. I was two weeks in and down 7 lbs. drinking Vanilla Hazelnut Kona coffee black and flavored unsweetened teas. Working through headaches and hunger, I was determined this was going to work. I read about Delay, Don't Deny Intermittent fasting shortly after the 7 lbs. lost were going up and down each day for weeks. I switched to plain black coffee, decaf green tea and lost another 10 lbs. in two weeks. No headaches and ravenous hunger as before with the flavored beverages. I've been clean fasting ever since. Thank you, Gin.
Temple BoClair	Having been a Yo-Yo dieter for more than 40 years, I was insulin resistant. Prior to June 2019 when I read DDD, I was a PROUD & DISCIPLINED 16:8 intermittent faster for 2 1/2 years. During each of my daily 16+ hour fasts I drank at least 2 liters of water. Additionally, I consistently indulged in sugar-free gum, mints & candies, hot lemon water, ACV water, Bullet-Proof Coffee (MCT Oil & Pure Irish Butter) or Coffee with 3 Tablespoons Heavy Whipping Cream & Stevia. After the 1st month & an initial 10 lbs. I never lost a single oz. of body fat, scale weight or clothing size. I know this because I was fanatical about weighing & tracking my progress on a digital scale & goal dress I'd purchased. Fast forward to June 12. My "AHA" moment came when Gin Stephens clearly explained the non-negotiable, SUPER-DUPER, UBER power of the CLEAN FAST. I heard, listened (& re-listened 3X), read (& re-read 3Xs), understood, then received the reasons why my IF experience was unsuccessful. I had unknowingly violated the 1st LAW of DDD. The rule of FASTING CLEAN! When I ignorantly added the no calorie, no sugar, no carbohydrate consumables to my fasts, I had constantly kept my insulin spiked, stalled my healing & hindered any further success or progess. Since then, I have successfully documented 133 squeaky CLEAN FASTS, released 15 lbs. & down-sized clothing 3 times. During which time I have consumed ABSOLUTELY NOTHING but filtered water, black coffee & PLAIN sparkling water. For me, the CLEAN FAST is an indisputable, undeniable TRUTH.

cont.

Tetesa Baker	I started intermitting fasting 16:8 every day. I did not change how I ate, I only wanted to focus on fasting to get the habit perfected! I loved it! I still had cream in my coffee and chewed gum every day! I read an article that said it was called dirty fasting and that it was ok! Did I lose weight? Sure did! Did I struggle? Sure did!! I was hungry all the time! When I read about Delay, Don't Deny intermittent fasting and learned about the clean fast, everything changed! I really didn't know that I had been spiking my insulin all day long!! From that day forth my fasts got easier! I was able to fast longer! Appetite correction happened and I knew my relationship with food would be changed forever.
Zoe from Nottinghamshire UK	Clean fasting does, for me, exactly what it says on the tin. I feel clean —internally. Unencumbered. Free. Once my window is closed, it feels so good for me not to think about food until my window is open. This doesn't mean I don't plan—I do, you have to plan, especially if you want to eat the good stuff! And oh boy—do you want to eat the good stuff!!! If I've only got a small window to eat and fuel my body, then I want the premium stuff that lasts and helps me through my next fasting closed window. The times when I've done the dirty fasting I've just felt off all day. Constantly hungry. I did the 5:2 routine back in 2015 where I had 500 calories a day—oh wow—that was SO hard! Once I start eating I find it very difficult to stop at that prescribed amount. For me, it is so much easier to clean fast, (water, black coffee, black tea) than to dirty fast. Another thing I find, is that for me, usually when my window is closed I can prepare food for me to eat either later, or for my family (Partner and 2 small children plus various pets) and I am not bothered by it. When my window is closed, it's closed! No ifs, buts, or maybes, or just one bite won't hurt . . . no way! It's closed! I am officially free from thinking about food. I have so much more mental availability for dealing with everything else!
Margo Kohlhoff	When I first started intermittent fasting, I was doing it on my own with just the concept of not eating for "x" hours and eating for "x" hours. I hadn't read any books or done much research at that point, but figured it would be easy to do. I did initially lose some weight slowly doing a dirty fast of flavored waters, or tea with some Stevia in it, or some other zero calorie drink, but it was always a struggle to get through the day. I couldn't wait for my eating window to open so I could EAT! After reading Gin's first book, I realized that the reason it was so hard for me to fast all day was because I wasn't REALLY fasting at all. Yes, I wasn't eating, but I wasn't clean fasting. I immediately switched to a clean fast of only water or plain sparkling water (I'm not a coffee drinker so I didn't have that hurdle to get over), and it was SO much easier to go all day with no hunger. I wasn't white knuckling it to get to my eating window, and thinking about eating all day. Once I began clean fasting, the weight seemed to come off more easily, and I didn't bounce back and forth on the scale. But, the best part of it was that it was so much easier to fast when I did it cleanly.

Cynthia Morrison Eike	Stopped using a breath spray (with artificial sweeteners) after 3 months into IF and ravenous hunger disappeared, making one meal a day much easier to keep!
Carrie Pinchuk, Aurora, IL	When I had zero calorie beverages and gum during my fast, I had to really push through. Once I understood clean fasting, I switched to plain, still water and black coffee during my fast and it was like a lightbulb went on. "Oh! I don't have to struggle." It really is easier to fast clean!
Marie McElroy	When I started IF, I continued drinking flavored coffee (not sweetened) thinking it wouldn't really matter. I was already in pretty good shape and only had a few pounds to lose. I convinced myself that I wasn't like those people who needed drastic changes. After a few months, I decided to follow Gin's advice and do it right!! I've been doing clean fasts for months now and the difference is real. I feel better, my skin and hair look better and I can totally tell that my body is functioning really well. At 67 I am at my goal weight, eat dessert when I want, and am way more active than most people much younger. The clean fast really made a difference!
Ali from Elk Grove	I started my IF journey before I read Gin's books. I had read online that zero calorie drinks were ok, so all during my "fast" I was drinking diet soda. I was hungry the whole time—constantly checking the time to see if it was time to open my window. I never made it past a 16-hour fast. Since finding Gin's books and online support groups I have been clean fasting, and it's EASY! I do anywhere from 20:4 to 23:1 without feeling hungry/deprived. My weight started dropping faster too! The clean fast is essential to sustaining this WOL!
Linnea Murray	I did IF for 6 years before learning about the clean fast. Fasting clean made it so much easier for me! I only drink water while fasting now and it's a breeze!
Sarah Adams	I was fasting clean for months but still struggling with finding the black coffee that wouldn't make me gag. Everyone says I would eventually like it so I just kept trying new brew/brands/temps etc. I finally found an iced coffee (black/unsweetened on the label) in the grocery store that was delish!! Home free!!! Skip to 3 weeks later . . . texting my IF friend my struggle for a few weeks with not being able to make my fast longer than 14 hours every day because I was so stinking hungry!! We went through all of the products that I have been having during my fast and reading labels. That wonderful "black/unsweetened" coffee that I have been thoroughly enjoying for 3 weeks? Ingredients say "natural flavoring." That's just IF speak for DIRTY!! Stopped drinking it immediately and easily went to my goal fast the next day. Moral of the story: ALWAYS READ THE INGREDIENTS.
Sheri from Alabama	When I first started IF in 2015, the general consensus was that you could use non-caloric sweeteners and flavors during the fast. I drank stevia coffee, flavored zero calorie drinks etc.

cont.

While I was able to lose weight, I white knuckled my fasts to 16 hours every day. Trying to reach 19 hours felt impossible. Then 20 months into my fasting journey, I found Gin and embraced the clean fast methodology.

Wow! Not only was I no longer white knuckling my fasts, I didn't have to restrict calories in my eating window and some weight creep that I was dealing with was reversed. After the inception of clean fasting, I had to actually go through the fat adaptation process, which confirms that when we don't clean fast, we don't become fat adapted. After 10 weeks of clean fasting, I lost the weight creep, and lost several more pounds with it.

Over the next year I witnessed astonishing changes to my body. Even though my weight remained constant at my goal weight, I went from having a soft squishy body, to a firm and lean body. Truly getting into the deep, clean fast allows my body to ramp up human growth hormone and autophagy. At the age of 46 my body looks the best it's every looked in my entire adult life.

The clean fast makes ALL the difference.

Debbie from Arizona	I had been clean fasting for a few months and was surprised, after an initial adjustment period, how easy it was to go all day without eating. I did struggle with the bitter taste of black coffee in the morning however, and so one day experimented with a pinch of cinnamon, fennel, and anise in my coffee prior to brewing. I was excited because this produced a less bitter cup of coffee but with no spice flavor. So I started using the spices every day in my brewed coffee. Over time, I began to struggle getting through the day without eating, to the point where eventually it was miserable. I even wondered what the heck; it used to be so easy. And then one day it hit me. I omitted the spices from the coffee just to see, and guess what? I fasted that day with no hunger. Amazing! Thank you so much Gin for the gift of not budging on the clean fast. It is powerful and it makes a monumental difference.
Jennifer Stoffer	Clean fasting makes such a difference. You feel so much better and tend not to overload once your window opens. It helps with clarity and no mid-day or late afternoon lags. Clean fasting has made such an improvement in maintaining this lifestyle. I never drank black coffee before but now I prefer it. Fast on y'all.
Tracy Bratton	A year before I knew about clean fasting I tried IF the dirty way. I couldn't stick to it. I drank a little cream in my coffee and diet soda all day long and then ate at night. I found it very hard to stick with this long term as I was having headaches, hunger pangs, and was just plain hangry. So after few weeks I gave up. After reading Gin's book and learning about fasting clean I made a commitment to try to clean fast 16-24 hrs each day. I have never felt better and I have lost 23 pounds since May 20. IF is so much easier and less stressful on the body if you just fast clean. (It did take a bit to get used to black coffee. I feel like a true grown-up now.)

Christie K from Decatur, GA	I was one of those people that had been pseudo-fasting for most of my younger years without realizing it or having a name for it. I just wasn't hungry and felt good when I waited a while to eat. After two pregnancies and breastfeeding, I picked up a diet soda habit because it was zero calories. (I mean sometimes six cans a day!) When I tried to get back to those longer breaks between meals, wow, it was so much harder than before. No body changes and a lot more hunger. After months of trying, I gave up. Finally learned about IF and the clean fast and cut out diet soda. Life and IF got SO much easier! Twenty-one lbs. off and my auto-immune craziness hasn't made a showing in the seven months I've been clean fasting! It's magic.
Danna from Sweden	I have been skipping breakfast and most lunches since my early teens, so over 17 years. I was, however, always chewing gum, having soda, and using cough drops. I kept gaining until I ballooned to 240 lbs. even though I was eating less than 500 calories half the time. A friend told me she lost weight on one meal a day and I couldn't understand why I just kept gaining doing the same thing. I delved into research and found Gin's clean fasting concept and I managed to lose over 35 lbs. and fasting has been effortless since.

Those stories are powerful, aren't they? Now that you understand the importance of the clean fast, it's time to learn some of the most popular approaches to intermittent fasting!

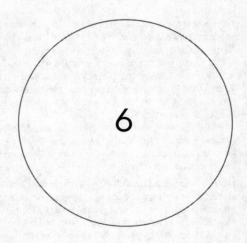

6

TIME-RESTRICTED EATING: AN "EATING WINDOW" APPROACH

One of the most popular intermittent fasting methods is time-restricted eating (TRE), which is casually referred to in the intermittent fasting community as an *eating window* approach. You'll usually hear the terminology *time-restricted feeding* (or TRF) if you're reading scientific journal articles about this IF strategy, but many of us who live the IF lifestyle prefer the sound of *time-restricted eating* over *time-restricted feeding*. After all, we aren't rats in a feeding study.

How does time-restricted eating work? It's pretty simple! With this approach to IF, there's literally nothing to count except time! You decide on the length of your eating window, and all foods you eat should be within that window. During this eating window, you choose the foods that work well for your body and make you feel great. (More about *how* to do this in the Feast section of the book!) During the fasting period, you fast clean, following the guidelines I explained to you in the previous two chapters.

Every day, your eating window "opens" with the first bite of food or sip of non-clean-fast-approved beverage. Once your window is open, you eat and drink according to your preferences. When you have had your last bite of food (or your last sip of non-clean-fast-approved beverage) for the day, you consider your eating window as closed, and the next fast begins. Get it? Fast. Feast. Repeat!

Many people wonder: Are you expected to eat constantly within your eating window? The answer is no. When your eating window is open, you have the *opportunity* to eat and drink, but that doesn't mean it's expected (or even beneficial) to eat nonstop. Don't worry about that yet; I'll explain more about choosing what and how much to eat in the Feast section of the book!

When you start exploring the various options for configuring your eating window, you may get confused with all the abbreviations and lingo—16:8? 19:5? 20:4? 23:1? OMAD? What's the difference, and what the heck do all these numbers and abbreviations mean?

Let me explain. Every day has twenty-four hours, and within each twenty-four-hour period, you will spend part of it fasting and part of it feasting. When we write the timing, we show it as a set of two numbers that add up to twenty-four. We first write the length of the daily *fast*, and then write the length of the daily *feast*. So, if you are doing a 16:8 protocol, then you would be fasting for sixteen hours a day and feasting for eight. With 20:4, you would fast for twenty hours and feast for four hours. With 23:1, you fast for twenty-three hours and have one hour of feasting. So, what's OMAD? That is an abbreviation for *one meal a day,* and it's a very popular form of TRE. It's the strategy that I use personally, and it works very well for me.

I want to caution you not to let all these possibilities overwhelm you! We are just *learning* about these variations for now. When you are ready to get started, you're going to follow the recommendations

I have laid out in the FAST Start chapter (chapter 10) to decide where to begin, and you'll select a pace that is just right for *you*. For now, though, let's get into the ins and outs of different eating window lengths so you can consider which ones you would like to experiment with after your FAST Start!

When we consider the spectrum of different eating window lengths, it's important to remember *why* we are fasting. We all want to experience the health benefits of IF, but most of us also want to ignite our fat-burning superpower.

To design an IF lifestyle that will give you the benefits you are looking for, you have to remember how an intermittent fasting lifestyle helps us access our stored fat for fuel:

- First, we deplete stored liver glycogen over time.

- Then, we flip the metabolic switch and transition to fat burning during the fast.

But two things must happen:

- You must fast sufficiently to deplete your stored liver glycogen.

- You can't eat so much food that you totally refill your liver glycogen every day or, even worse, store excess food away as new fat.

While IF may contain a degree of hormonal and metabolic "magic," it's not so magical that you can overeat in your eating window and expect to see weight loss. You may still see health benefits, of course.

Before I explain a variety of TRE approaches, I want you to keep this in the back of your mind: the fat-burning benefits generally begin somewhere between the twelve- and sixteen-hour mark, though they really ramp up between hours eighteen and twenty-four. Also, insulin goes down dramatically within the first twenty-four hours of fasting; in a 1993 study, researchers found that insulin levels go down by approximately 50 percent overall between hours twelve and seventy-two of fasting, while 70 percent of that overall decrease happened in the first twenty-four hours.[1] All of this together indicates that the fat-burning sweet spot of fasting for most people may be found within that eighteen- to twenty-four-hour fasting period.

So, as you read about the various options, think about how each may help you reach your personal goals:

- If you are fasting for health purposes only and don't want to lose any weight, you'll select an approach that has a shorter fasting period, such as 12:12 or 16:8 (or something in between).

- If fat loss is your main goal, you'll likely want to have a longer daily fast to make sure you experience that fat-burning sweet spot—19:5, 20:4, 23:1, and OMAD are all great options!

POPULAR TRE / EATING WINDOW OPTIONS

Arranged in order from longest eating window to shortest eating window.

12:12

The consensus is that the health benefits of TRE begin with something as generous as a 12:12 approach. As I've already mentioned, the fat-burning benefits generally begin between the twelve- and sixteen-hour mark, though they really ramp up between hours eighteen and twenty-four. So, if fat burning is your goal, you want to structure your approach so that you get into the fat-burning zone, which 12:12 won't accomplish; 12:12 isn't very different from a typical three-meals-a-day eating pattern, so you are unlikely to see much weight loss with this approach—but it is a place to start. When you decide to follow a 12:12 approach, it may be as simple as eliminating your current late-night eating habits, and BOOM! You're doing it. That doesn't sound so hard, does it?

cont.

Sample 12:12 schedules:

7:00 a.m.–7:00 p.m.: Breakfast at 7:00 a.m., lunch midday, dinner finished by 7:00 p.m.

8:00 a.m.–8:00 p.m.: Breakfast at 8:00 a.m., lunch midday, dinner finished by 8:00 p.m.

9:00 a.m.–9:00 p.m.: Breakfast at 9:00 a.m., lunch midday, dinner finished by 9:00 p.m.

16:8

With a 16:8 approach, you're fitting all your food intake into an eight-hour daily eating window. Usually, this is as simple as skipping one of your typical meals, and you're doing 16:8. Most people who choose 16:8 tend to skip breakfast, eat lunch and dinner, and close their window after dinner, though there are others who prefer to shift the window earlier and eat breakfast and lunch, skipping dinner each day.

The popularity of 16:8 skyrocketed in 2012 with the release of the book *The 8-Hour Diet*. I certainly tried it, with a great deal of enthusiasm! The subtitle really appealed to me: *Watch the Pounds Disappear Without Watching What You Eat!*

Sorry, y'all. I have to tell you the truth here.

You are probably not going to be able to "Watch the Pounds Disappear Without Watching What You Eat!" in an eating window of eight hours (and you may not even be able to do that in a shorter window). We will get into specifics of how to figure out the right *amount* and *types* of food for you in the Feast section of the book. Quantity (and quality) of food still matters, even with IF.

The truth of the matter is, when you have a longer eating window like this one, you have to be more mindful of what you eat and how much. Sixteen hours of fasting doesn't give you much time in the fat-burning zone, and you can do a lot of eating in eight hours. And if peak fat burning happens between hours eighteen and twenty-four of a fast, you can see that 16:8 would not quite get you there.

Both my (always slim) husband and my (always slim) son follow a loose 16:8 approach. Neither ever needed to lose any fat, and they started strictly for the health benefits. They both wake up and have black coffee and water in the morning, and then they open their eating window with lunch. Later, they have dinner. Easy-peasy.

Sample 16:8 schedules:
12:00 p.m.–8:00 p.m.: Lunch at 12:00 p.m., dinner finished by 8:00 p.m.
10:00 a.m.–6:00 p.m.: Brunch midday, dinner finished by 6:00 p.m.
9:00 a.m.–5:00 p.m.: Breakfast at 9:00 a.m., lunch midday, dinner finished by 5:00 p.m.

19:5

If you recall that fat burning begins to ramp up between hours twelve and sixteen and the fat-burning sweet spot for most people may be found within that eighteen- to twenty-four-hour fasting period, you can see how 19:5 is a great approach for many. You have time to flip the metabolic switch every day and spend somewhere between one and seven hours of your nineteen-hour fast in the fat-burning state, depending upon whether *you* start burning fat at hour twelve of the fast or at hour eighteen of the fast, or somewhere in between.

The 19:5 approach was my personal weight-loss sweet spot, and I first started experimenting with it in around 2009. I never really embraced IF as a lifestyle until 2014, however, so I never could make it stick until I changed my mind-set. More about the importance of this concept in the mind-set chapter (found in the Repeat section of the book!).

My introduction to 19:5 came from a book called *The Fast-5 Diet and the Fast-5 Lifestyle,* written by Dr. Bert Herring. When I stuck consistently to the 19:5 plan, I saw slow and steady weight loss of about a pound per week. That doesn't mean that *you* will have this same result from 19:5, of course. You'll need to tweak and experiment to find *your* ideal approach.

cont.

Sample 19:5 schedules:

5:00 p.m.–10:00 p.m.: Begin eating at 5:00 p.m., with all food for the day finished by 10:00 p.m.

Note: This is the original eating window proposed by Dr. Herring in his *Fast-5* book and the one he personally follows.

12:00 p.m.–5:00 p.m.: Lunch at 12:00 p.m., dinner finished by 5:00 p.m.

2:00 p.m.–7:00 p.m.: Afternoon snack at 2:00 p.m., dinner finished by 7:00 p.m.

8:00 a.m.–1:00 p.m.: Breakfast at 8:00 a.m., lunch finished by 1:00 p.m.

OMAD: "One Meal a Day"

The concept of only eating one meal a day might sound overly restrictive, but that's far from the truth! It's actually a very flexible and enjoyable way to live.

What is OMAD? First, think about the typical eating pattern for most people: breakfast, lunch, and dinner, or three meals per day. When you follow OMAD, you are eating only one actual *meal* per day, so you'll choose breakfast, lunch, or dinner as your one main meal of the day. This doesn't mean you are limited to one *plate* of food or that you have to eat it within one hour. After all, this approach isn't called OPAD (one plate a day) or OHAD (one hour a day, or 23:1).

I consider myself to be an OMADer, and I generally eat within an eating window of two to five hours per day, meaning that my OMAD fits into a TRE window somewhere between 22:2 and 19:5.

You may be shaking your head at this point. How could a two- to five-hour eating window possibly be OMAD?

I like to compare what I do to fine dining. If I went to a restaurant for dinner, we would probably start with an appetizer course. Next, I would have a salad, followed by the entrée and some sort of dessert. The way I approach my OMAD eating window is very similar to the amount of food from this type of restaurant meal. I generally open my window with something akin to an appetizer. An hour or two later, I usually have my main meal. After dinner, I might finish my glass of wine while I spend some time with my husband.

To close my eating window, I'll often have something sweet or even a little cheese. As you see from this example, I eat one actual meal most days, and I eat it at a pace that fits into my daily schedule.

There are some purists out there who think if you're eating more than one plate of food or if your window lasts longer than one hour, you're not doing OMAD, but I disagree, and so do scientists. In a 2007 study with human subjects, a team of scientists compared what they called a "1 meal per day diet" with the typical eating pattern of three meals per day.[2] In their study, the "1 meal per day diet" group ate within a four-hour period each day, giving them a minimum daily fast of twenty hours.

This was actually a pretty cool study; the participants eating OMAD were given the same number of calories and a similar meal nutrient composition as those eating three meals a day (this worked out to an average of 2,396 calories per day). The calorie intake was designed to result in weight maintenance rather than weight loss, but even so, the OMAD group lost 2.1 kg of body fat and gained 0.7 kg of muscle mass (while those in the three-meal group didn't see significant differences). So, even though all the participants ate the equivalent of a whole day's worth of food, those who ate it within a four-hour period lost fat and gained muscle during the short eight-week study period. Imagine what might have happened if they had not been forced to eat a whole day's worth of food within their one-meal period!

Luckily, we don't have to imagine it; in a 2015 study, mice who were fed 70 percent of their normal food intake once a day had significantly less fat than their non-fasting mouse friends. The muscle mass of both groups was similar, but as they got older, the mice fed once a day didn't have the typical age-related loss of muscle mass usually seen in aging mice. They also had significantly *higher* bone densities than the other mice, and their fasting insulin levels were significantly lower.[3] (While this particular study didn't report how long it took the mice to eat the food they were given, other studies on mice who were fed 70 percent of their normal food intake once a day found that they generally ate all their food within a two-hour period.)[4]

Based on these two studies, we can see that even if you eat a full day's

cont.

worth of food during your OMAD eating window, you should expect to see fat loss, but if you eat less food than you would typically eat over the course of a whole day, the benefits should be even more significant. Personally, I am certain that I don't eat as much food in my daily OMAD eating window as I would eat if I ate all day long, even though I eat enough food to make me feel not only satisfied but definitely not like I am on any kind of restrictive diet plan.

Sample OMAD schedules:

4:00 p.m.–9:00 p.m.: Appetizer at 4:00 p.m., main meal at 6:30 p.m., dessert finished by 9:00 p.m.

(This is very similar to the schedule that I follow most days. My eating window length may vary a bit from day to day, but this is how I generally structure my meal.)

8:00 a.m.–12:00 p.m.: Open window with a creamy coffee at 8:00 a.m., main meal finished by 12:00 p.m.

2:00 p.m.–5:00 p.m.: Main meal at 2:00 p.m., dessert finished by 5:00 p.m.

6:00 p.m.–7:00 p.m.: Main meal eaten between 6:00 p.m. and 7:00 p.m.

Notice that each of these sample OMAD schedules varies in window length. Never forget that OMAD is a flexible concept! As long as you are eating one actual meal within an eating window that works for you, you're doing OMAD Gin-style.

23:1

This is the most extreme daily-eating-window approach, but some people absolutely love the simplicity of having a one-hour eating window. You open your window, you eat, and then you close it.

One concern with long-term 23:1 is that you may tend to eat the same amount of food from day to day and your body may adapt to your eating pattern. It's true; even though IF is protective of metabolism in general, the body also tends to adapt to anything that is the same day in and day out. On the flip side, the body is less likely to adapt when you vary the amount you eat from day to day.[5] If and when your body adapts to 23:1, you may stop losing weight, and you may even start getting increased hunger signals from your body. Never fear! If this happens, you'll know that it's time to shake things up with some longer eating windows (or try the up-and-down-day approach that I'll explain in the next chapter).

Sample 23:1 schedules:
6:00 p.m.–7:00 p.m.: Dinner between 6:00 p.m. and 7:00 p.m.
3:00 p.m.–4:00 p.m.: Early dinner between 3:00 p.m. and 4:00 p.m.
10:00 a.m.–11:00 a.m.: Large breakfast or early lunch between 10:00 a.m. and 11:00 a.m.

While these are some of the most popular approaches to TRE, keep in mind that these are not the only possibilities for how you can structure your eating window. You could choose any combination of fasting and feasting that works for you (14:10, 17:7, 20:4, 22:2, etc.). You also don't have to follow the same exact approach from day to day. One day you might be 19:5, and the next you might be 20:4, followed by a day of 16:8. Not only is that okay, but there may be some benefit to switching things up from day to day so your body doesn't become too comfortable with the same routine. Research shows that keeping your body guessing may prevent metabolic adaptation, which is always a good thing.[6]

When considering when to have your daily eating window, you may wonder if it's better to have an early eating window or if it's better to have it later in the day. While there is a train of thought among the scientists who study fasting that there may be benefits to an early eating window,[7] there are still no long-term studies directly comparing early eating windows to late eating windows, with all other factors being equal. Even though we don't yet have a long-term study, there is one short study from 2019 that compared an early eating window with a late eating window. Participants had a daily nine-hour eating window for one week, and they either ate from 8:00

a.m. to 5:00 p.m. or 12:00 p.m. to 9:00 p.m. Scientists found that participants had similar improvements in glycemic response, no matter which time of day they ate.[8] This was such a short study, however, so it will be interesting to see what results are found from longer studies in the future. Even these scientists who are interested in discovering the "best" time for a TRF schedule say that "future studies should also consider how an individual's own chronotype may impact the magnitude of responses when TRF is commenced early or late."[9] What they are saying here is that people may indeed have individual differences that mean there really is *not* a one-size-fits-all best time to structure your eating window!

Since we don't (yet) have conclusive scientific data comparing various eating window timings, let's look at what current intermittent fasters are doing while living their lives in the real world. In my online intermittent fasting community, I performed an unscientific and very informal survey, and this is what thousands of IFers from around the world reported:

Question: What have you found is the best time for you to have your eating window?

- 61 percent prefer an evening eating window

- 25 percent favor a midday eating window

- 2 percent choose a morning eating window

- 12 percent switch up the timing of their eating window from day to day

As you can see, there is no one eating window schedule that suits everyone!

The bottom line is this: I believe that the best eating window for you is the one that feels like a lifestyle you can stick with. You'll only know this by experimenting with different times. Don't try to force yourself to follow anyone else's preferred protocol; trust yourself to figure out what feels right to you!

Why do so many intermittent fasters absolutely love the daily-eating-window approach? Here are a few of the main reasons people love time-restricted eating:

- TRE is extremely flexible! You can adjust your eating window to fit any social event or situation you can imagine. Not only is it okay to change things up, it may provide metabolic benefits.

- With TRE, you have clear boundaries, which reduces daily decision fatigue. At any given moment, your window is either open or it's closed. If it's open, you eat. If it's closed, you don't. It's amazing how much peace you feel when every waking moment isn't consumed with decisions about whether you should or shouldn't be eating something.

- With TRE, you eat delicious food until you are satisfied every single day with no calorie counting required.

Are there any downsides to the daily-eating-window approach? Here are some of the things to keep in mind:

- TRE may be more of a maintenance lifestyle for some people. While eating all your food within a daily eating window provides numerous health benefits, not everyone loses weight following this approach.

- If you've been a dieter for a long time and have a slowed metabolism, TRE might not give you enough of a metabolic boost. If this describes you, you may need the metabolic boosting strategies from the up-and-down-day chapter (chapter 7).

- If you have been overweight or obese for decades, you likely have higher baseline levels of insulin. If this is true, TRE may not give your body enough fasting time to lower insulin levels. You may need some longer periods of fasting, such as those described in the up-and-down-day chapter (chapter 7).

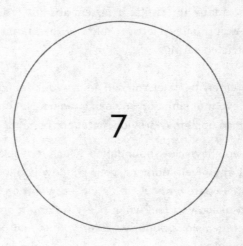

7

ALTERNATE-DAY FASTING PROTOCOLS: THE "UP-AND-DOWN-DAY" APPROACH

While time-restricted eating approaches to intermittent fasting are very popular, the daily-eating-window approach is not the only way to structure an IF protocol. In this chapter, I will explain the variety of alternate-day, or "up-and-down-day" approaches out there. 5:2? 4:3? ADF? What in the world do all these numbers and letters mean, and how can you apply these approaches to your life?

The concept of an up-and-down-day approach really took off in 2012, when British physician Dr. Michael Mosley appeared in a BBC program called *Eat, Fast, and Live Longer.* Based on the research of Dr. Krista Varady, who was studying an every-other-day fasting protocol at the University of Illinois, Dr. Mosley found that by restricting what he was eating on just two days of the week and eating "normally" on the other five days, he not only lost weight but also saw an improvement in various health markers. Following that broadcast, there was so much interest in the 5:2 protocol that Dr. Mosley coauthored a book to bring the plan to the world.

Before getting into the science behind these approaches and a discussion about who would benefit from this type of IF protocol, let's learn the lingo. When you see an up-and-down-day approach such as 5:2, notice that the two numbers add up to 7. The first number refers to how many days per week you eat "normally" (those are your "up" days), and the second number indicates how many days per week you "fast" (those are your "down" days).

So, you can see that a weekly 5:2 pattern has five up days and two down days. A 4:3 approach would have four up days and three down days. A 6:1 approach would have six up days and one down day. True ADF, or "alternate-daily fasting," requires that you literally alternate from day to day: up day, down day, up day, down day, and so on.

No matter which up-and-down-day plan you choose, there are two recommended options for how to structure your down days:

OPTION 1: 500-CALORIE DOWN DAYS

- If you choose this option, you will still be eating a small meal on the down days, and so this approach is frequently referred to as a "modified fast day."

- You'll wake up on the down day and stick to clean-fast-approved beverages throughout the day.

- At whichever point of the day that works for you, you'll eat one meal of up to 500 calories.

- Keep in mind that with this approach to a down day, you aren't doing a full fast, but you absolutely should fast clean before and after your one 500-calorie meal so that you maximize the benefits of the clean fast.

- In the Feast section of this book, I am going to explain why all calories aren't created equal, how there are many flaws to weight-loss approaches that rely on calorie counting, and that I don't generally recommend calorie counting as a useful strategy. For that reason, it may confuse you to see a recommendation here for a 500-calorie down day. Isn't this calorie counting? The key is that when you are attempting an up-and-down-day protocol, you need to ensure that your down day really is "down." Limiting yourself to 500 calories on down days is a great way to make sure you are accomplishing this goal. I promise this is the only time you'll have to count anything other than time!

Benefits of the 500-calorie option:

- You eat every day.

- You may find it is easier to sleep on a 500-calorie day than on a full-fast day.

Drawbacks to the 500-calorie option:

- Some people find that it is actually harder to limit food intake to 500 calories than it is to do a complete fast. Plus, counting calories is tedious.

- You have less time in the fully fasted state because you're eating that small meal.

OPTION 2: FULL FASTS OF 36 TO 42 HOURS

Before I get into details, there is one thing I want to make clear: sometimes, people think a fast of 36 to 42 hours is an extended fast (EF), but ADF is *not* actually the same as "extended fasting." While there is no official dictionary definition of extended fasting that I am aware of, to me, EFs are when you move *beyond* ADF territory. Extended fasts are something else entirely and are not within the scope of this book. More about why this is true in the chapter about fasting red flags.

So, now that that's out of the way, let's learn about the full-fast option for down days.

- If you choose this option, you won't eat at all because you're doing a full fast for approximately 36 to 42 hours.

- You'll wake up on the down day and stick to clean-fast-approved beverages all day.

- Then you'll go to bed without eating, knowing that when you wake up, it's an up day.

Benefits of the full-fast option:

- You have a longer period in the fasted state, which means that you'll have increased autophagy, more time with lowered insulin levels, and more time in the fat-burning state.

- Some people find that it is easier to do a full fast than to stop after a 500-calorie meal.

Drawbacks to the full-fast option:

- You may have so much energy (thanks to ketosis) that it is hard to sleep.

- It can be psychologically difficult to skip a whole day of eating, particularly at first.

•

Whether you choose the 500-calorie modified fast day or the 36- to 42-hour full fast, on the up days, you'll eat without restriction. While that doesn't mean that you should force-feed yourself or purposefully overeat just because you "can," you *do* want to be careful that you are not "dieting" or having a short eating window on any day following a down day.

This is *really important*, so I will say it again:

**On any up day that is directly following a down day,
do *not* purposefully restrict what you are eating or eat
within a short eating window.**

Why is this so important that I said it twice? Well, it has to do with the reason the up days are so important.

As I mentioned in earlier chapters, our bodies can adapt to under-eating over time. Even with IF, which provides a distinct metabolic and hormonal advantage over a traditional low-calorie plan, you may still see some metabolic adaptation over time if you over-restrict for a prolonged period or keep the amount you eat consistent from day to day. But as I've already told you in the previous chapter, we have research that teaches us that the body is less likely to adapt when you vary the amount you eat from day to day.[1]

What *really* keeps the metabolism revved up and humming along? Overfeeding! In one study, scientists found that participants saw a 7 percent boost in metabolic rate following a three-day over-feeding period.[2] They also had a 28 percent increase in leptin, which is the satiety hormone. (It's interesting to note that the boost was seen when the participants ate excess carbohydrates, but not when they ate excess fat.) In another study, sixteen lean people were over-fed by one thousand excess calories per day.[3] Over this eight-week study, the participants' basal metabolic rates (BMRs) increased rap-idly in response to the overfeeding before going back down and then leveling off (at a point that was higher than their initial BMR values). Leptin levels also went up in this study.

Once you understand this, you will want to fully embrace the "up" nature of your up days: these up-and-down-day protocols work so well *because* of this day-to-day variability between the up and the down days. For that reason, the last thing you want to do is over-restrict on your up days. In an early ADF study, scientists reported that the participants ate an average of 100–110 percent of their body's calculated "energy needs" on the up days.[4] Yep! In that study, many of them were "overfeeding" by eating above their bodies' maintenance levels and none of them were "dieting" in any way on their up days! An up day should contain *at least* two to three meals in a *minimum* of a six- to eight-hour period. It's perfectly fine to follow a typical three-meal-a-day eating pattern on your up days, as you should absolutely not be "dieting" in any way on up days!

So, knowing what we know now, we could predict that restricting food intake on the up days could have a detrimental long-term effect. While we might have quicker initial weight loss, we would miss out on the metabolic-boosting effect of a true up day. On an up day, eat! Even if you end up eating more food than your body needs, as long as you aren't stuffing yourself silly, the up days will be balanced out by the down days. You'll have the fat-loss benefits of the down days coupled with the metabolic boosting benefits of the up days.

Besides the fat loss and metabolic benefits of an up-and-down-day protocol, there are also body composition benefits. We have already learned that fasting helps us flip the metabolic switch, allowing us to harness our fat-burning superpowers while retaining muscle mass. So, we would expect studies on ADF to show this. That's exactly what a 2016 scientific review found![5] Scientists looked at all the studies conducted using human subjects that compared ADF protocols to traditional low-calorie dieting, and their meta-analysis found that while the subjects on a low-calorie diet lost more overall scale weight than the ADFers, the ADF subjects lost more fat and retained more muscle than the low-calorie dieters. This is such a foundational concept to understand; the ADFers lost more fat and retained more muscle than those following a traditional low-calorie diet, even though they lost less scale weight! This is an example of what we in the IF world call *body recomposition*.

What does this mean for us? Well, with ADF, we may not see results as quickly on the scale as we would with a typical low-calorie diet, but we *will* see our bodies shrink in size! How does this happen? One pound of fat takes up more space than one pound of muscle, so someone who loses a pound of fat but gains a pound of muscle will still weigh the same but will be visibly smaller in size and leaner.

Now that we understand how these up and down days work, let's discuss who would benefit the most from an up-and-down-day protocol. The up-and-down-day approach is highly recommended:

- *If you have insulin resistance.* The down days (particularly if you choose the full-fast option) are great for reducing your insulin levels.

- *If you are dealing with metabolic slowdown.* The up days come with a metabolic-boosting benefit that your body may need.

- *If you have plateaued while using an eating-window approach.* If you find that your body adapts to the regularity of a daily eating window, the up-and-down-day pattern is great for shaking things up and getting weight loss moving in the right direction.

Keep this in mind: if you're doing well on an eating-window approach and you enjoy it, there is no need for you to experiment with an up-and-down-day protocol unless you want to. But who knows? You might try it and absolutely love it! I know plenty of IFers who do. I also know many IFers who view the up-and-down-day protocols as a temporary intervention that they need to do for a time, and they plan to return to the eating-window approach eventually for their permanent IF lifestyle.

So, which approach to try? 5:2? 4:3? True ADF? Let's look at each of these individually and discuss who would benefit from each.

5:2

Five up days / Two down days

A 5:2 plan fits easily into a week, and it provides both flexibility and predictability. When I tried 5:2, I chose my two down days each week to occur on days when I knew I would be less likely to have social obligations. For me, that was Monday and Thursday. Every Monday and Thursday were down days, and I experimented with both the 500-calorie and the full-fast options. Personally, the full-fast option was easier for me, because I am the kind of person who enjoys eating a hearty meal; limiting myself to 500 calories was harder than doing a full fast. Does that mean a full fast is universally "better"? No! Experiment to see which option feels better to you, and feel confident that either approach is going to provide the benefits of a down day.

Is there something magical about choosing Monday and Thursday as down days? Of course not! Choose the days that work best for your schedule. If I knew that I had a social event on a Thursday, it was easy to shift my down day to a different day, such as Wednesday or Friday.

When I did 5:2, it was easy to choose two down days during the week and then have complete freedom and flexibility over the weekend. I loved knowing that I could eat whenever I wanted on Friday, Saturday, and Sunday each week.

One thing I want to emphasize: 5:2 may or may not be a weight-loss protocol for you. While there are definitely health benefits to this approach, two down days per week may not be sufficient for weight loss. That was certainly true for me; 5:2 was a great maintenance protocol for my body. For weight loss, I needed 4:3.

4:3

Four up days / Three down days

Just as with 5:2, 4:3 also fits easily into a week and provides both flexibility and predictability. When I used the 4:3 approach, I selected down days that would work best with my schedule, and that meant that my usual down days were Sunday, Tuesday, and Thursday. I was always ready to get back to a down day on Sunday after eating freely on Friday and Saturday!

As with 5:2, you can adjust your schedule to fit your social events. If I knew that I had a social event on a Sunday, I could easily shift my down days for that week. Most weeks, though, I stuck with the predictability of Sunday, Tuesday, and Thursday.

cont.

4:3 was a great weight-loss protocol for my body. When I followed it, I lost at the rate of about a pound per week. (More about my recommendations for effectively tracking your progress in the Repeat section of the book!)

ADF

Alternate-daily fasting

ADF means that you alternate up and down days, so each week is going to be different. One week you will fast on Sunday, Tuesday, Thursday, and Saturday, and the next week you fast on Monday, Wednesday, and Friday. While each week is different (and therefore unpredictable), the *rhythm* of up-down-up-down is something many ADFers really enjoy.

While true ADF is less flexible than either 5:2 or 4:3, you can make a shift here and there for special occasions. If, for example, a special event is scheduled for a day that should be a down day for you, you can always have a second up day and then get right back into the down-and-up pattern. What you don't want to do is schedule two down days in a row; remember that up ALWAYS follows down!

Whether you choose 5:2, 4:3, or ADF, always remember this: no matter which form of up-and-down-day fasting you pick, make sure to have a true up day after *every* down day. You shouldn't schedule two down days in a row or have one down day and then have one meal on the following day. This isn't the fasting Olympics, where the more you can fast, the better it is. Never forget that we need the up pattern to balance out the down. I really want to hammer that last point home; the key to the whole thing is the *up* day following *every* down day. That's the part that lets your body know you are not in danger of starving. That's the part that keeps our metabolisms humming along.

So, please do not do an ADF pattern where you do a full fast for 46 to 48 hours, eat one meal, and then start another 46- to 48-hour fast. That is *not* ADF, and it is *not* recommended.

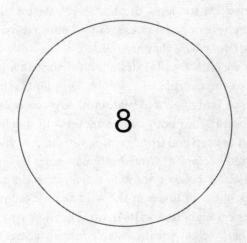

8

YOUR INTERMITTENT FASTING TOOLBOX

Now that you have learned about the main approaches to IF (eating windows versus up-and-down days), I will teach you how to combine these various intermittent fasting strategies to create a truly individualized and customizable intermittent fasting program. I want you to think of all these approaches as your IF toolbox, and I want you to understand how (and when!) to switch things up!

First, you may be wondering why we would *need* to switch things up. Let's learn about a very important protective mechanism in the body called *homeostasis*.

Within our bodies, we have systems in place to ensure we maintain an environment that remains within certain ranges. Body temperature is one example of this concept, as is blood glucose level, fluid balance, and so on. To put it into simple terms, when something gets out of whack, the body has mechanisms in place to bring it back into balance. If we overheat, we sweat to bring down our temperatures.

If blood glucose gets too high, our bodies release insulin to lower it. When we exercise, our heart rates go up to pump oxygen and nutrients to the muscles where they are needed.

Our body weights are also designed to work this way. I'm sure you've heard of the concept of a weight "set point." This refers to a weight that your body fights to maintain. Are you over your body's preferred set point? Your body can crank up your metabolic rate and increase leptin to keep you from gaining weight. Are you under your body's preferred set point? Your body can turn *down* your metabolic rate and also increase ghrelin to drive you to eat more and gain weight.[1] Think about animals in the wild as an example. Have you ever seen an overweight lion in its natural habitat? Animals manage to maintain their weight within a stable range without counting the first calorie or hiring a physical trainer. It's only when animals are in captivity, being fed by humans, or domesticated that we see them start gaining weight beyond their normal range.

If we were all still eating real foods that we had to gather or hunt for ourselves, eating only until satisfied, and remaining physically active as we went about the strenuous tasks of staying alive, we wouldn't have weight problems, either. But we eat highly processed foods. We are taught to clean our plates and reward ourselves with food. Our homes are filled with labor-saving devices. As a result, our natural weight control mechanisms become "broken," and we end up with the current obesity epidemic.

As I have already explained in previous chapters, intermittent fasting is a great way to "fix" much of what has become broken. We lower insulin levels, allowing us to tap into stored fat. Our bodies ignite our natural fat-burning superpower, our metabolic rates are protected to some degree, we build muscle thanks to increased human growth hormone, and our leptin and ghrelin get back into balance, just as nature intended!

Except for one thing: our bodies *still* have that pesky tendency to maintain homeostasis. Sigh.

This means that even when you are an intermittent faster, you will likely need to actively work against your body's natural tendencies to settle at a weight where *it's* happy but *you're* not.

First, before I give the mistaken idea that weight loss is hopeless, don't despair. The good news is that I believe that we *can* lower our bodies' set points over time. Of course, if we knew exactly *how* to lower our set points, we would all do it, and BAM! Obesity eradicated! Unfortunately, the science around the theory of the weight set point is still murky. Fortunately, some research suggests that if you can maintain weight loss for a year, your body is likely to "accept" the new weight as your new set point.[2] That certainly seems to be true for me; I have maintained my weight within a tight range for over five years now (even as my body goes through menopause), and I don't count a single calorie or consciously restrict what I'm eating. I haven't gotten on a scale in over three years, and I am still able to wear all my favorite clothes, season after season. I am confident that intermittent fasting has allowed me to "reset" my body's set point.

Still, however, you must lose the weight you want (and need) to lose; nobody wants to end up stuck at a set point that is higher than the weight that is healthy for their bodies. The good news is that when we *understand* homeostasis, we are better equipped to fight against it.

As I've already mentioned in both the eating window chapter and the up-and-down-day chapter, your body is less likely to adapt when you switch things up from day to day.[3] That's where your intermittent fasting toolbox comes in handy!

There's one easy rule that you should follow:

Switching things up from time to time is a great idea.

See! I told you it was an easy rule.

What does this look like in practice? It means that you can mix and match, selecting from all the available intermittent fasting strategies to purposefully switch things up. It also means that you can keep a close eye on your results over time, and if you see that your progress is slowing down, you'll know that it's time to pull another tool out of your toolbox.

TOOLBOX STRATEGY 1:
SWITCH YOUR IF APPROACH COMPLETELY

This one is pretty simple; if you have been following the eating-window approach, switch to an up-and-down-day approach for a few weeks. If you've been following the up-and-down-day approach, switch to an eating-window approach for a few weeks. This strategy is so simple, in fact, that you don't even need a diagram to see how it would look.

TOOLBOX STRATEGY 2:
ALTERNATE EATING-WINDOW LENGTHS

This approach creates a loose version of up-and-down days (which should keep your body guessing), but the appeal is that you don't have to count calories or have a full fast for a down day!

In this sample week, there are three days of 23:1, where you are likely to consume less food simply due to the nature of the one-hour eating window. While they aren't true down days in the sense that you are restricting yourself to 500 calories or doing a full fast, the varying schedule gives you a subtle up-and-down pattern that should provide benefits.

MONDAY	TUESDAY	WEDNESDAY	THURSDAY	FRIDAY	SATURDAY	SUNDAY
23:1	18:6	23:1	18:6	23:1	16:8	19:5

TOOLBOX STRATEGY 3:
CREATE A HYBRID APPROACH

Good news! You don't have to choose one IF approach over the other! Instead, you can create a hybrid approach where you have some down days, some up days, and then some other days with eating windows. This means that IF can be totally customizable to fit into your schedule and work around life's special events!

Let's look at a couple of examples of how this might look in practice.

In this first hybrid-approach sample schedule, you're doing a modified 6:1 (one down day followed by one up day) while also switching up eating-window lengths throughout the week. As you can imagine, this would be a great way to structure your week if you tend to have special events on Saturdays.

MONDAY	TUESDAY	WEDNESDAY	THURSDAY	FRIDAY	SATURDAY	SUNDAY
20:4	19:5	20:4	18:6	Down day	Up day	19:5
4-hour eating window	5-hour eating window	4-hour eating window	6-hour eating window	500-calorie down day or full fast	6- to 12-hour eating window (eat at least two meals, since any day after a down day should be a true up day!)	5-hour eating window

In this second hybrid-approach example, you are combining 5:2 with 19:5. In this sample week, there are two down days, two up days (never forget that an up day should always follow a down day!), and then the other three days are 19:5. This gives you the fat-burning power of a couple of down days, the metabolic boost of a couple of up days, and the ease of a few 19:5 days.

MONDAY	TUESDAY	WEDNESDAY	THURSDAY	FRIDAY	SATURDAY	SUNDAY
Down day	Up day	19:5	Down day	Up day	19:5	19:5
500-calorie down day or full fast	6- to 12-hour eating window (eat at least two meals, since any day after a down day should be a true up day!)	5-hour eating window	500-calorie down day or full fast	6- to 12-hour eating window (eat at least two meals, since any day after a down day should be a true up day!)	5-hour eating window	5-hour eating window

The three toolbox strategies that I just described are by no means the only ways you can structure your IF protocol. Remember what I told you in the Welcome for the book: *you* are in charge! So, always keep in mind that *you* have the freedom to design your own IF lifestyle! You have all the tools you need, and you have permission to experiment!

When deciding how to switch things up, it can be helpful to think about your current goals. If you are trying to lose weight, you want to maximize fat burning. In that case, arrange your schedule with more down days (never forgetting that every down day should be followed by a true up day!) and have fewer days with longer eating windows. If weight maintenance is your goal, you would choose fewer down days and have longer eating windows.

Here's some really good news! Over time, you'll find that you begin to adjust what you're doing effortlessly as you live your life. Some days, you'll be busy and end up with a shorter eating window. Then the next day, you may find that you get hungry earlier in the day and need a longer eating window. This is very much how it looks for me. I listen to my body and adjust accordingly. Last week, I went on vacation for a few days. As a result, I had some longer eating windows. When I got back home, my body naturally didn't want as much food for a few days. *That,* my friends, is true freedom. I no longer count hours or plan my eating windows at all; I simply live my life. I think that's the best toolbox of all; it's the one that is truly effortless and requires no thought!

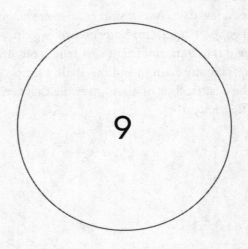

JUST SAY NO:
FASTING RED FLAGS

Now that we have fully stocked our IF toolbox, it's time for a word of caution. Our goal is to always be safe when living an intermittent fasting lifestyle. There are certain red flags that you need to be aware of, so let's explore each of these in detail. Pay attention to these red flags, and make sure that you're always making safe decisions for your specific situation.

RED FLAG ONE: OVER-FASTING

We live in a world where "more" is often considered to be "better." You want to run? Try marathons! If that isn't enough of a challenge for you, now we have ultramarathons. What's next? Super-de-duper-megathons?

Rather than running marathons, ultramarathons, or super-de-duper-megathons, most of us are better off sticking to a gentler exercise plan, and we know that about ourselves. By the way, while there is nothing wrong with physically challenging yourself if you feel great doing so, research shows that adult sports injuries are increasing due to both an uptick in the popularity of these activities and also the increased intensity of today's training routines.[1] Many of these injuries are related to overuse, and one problem is when we try to do too much, too soon, without building up to it. Another problem comes when we don't give our bodies time to rest and recover from intense exercise.

We can apply this same concept from exercise to intermittent fasting. Just as we need to build up to a more intense exercise plan, we need to give our bodies time to adjust to fasting. And just as athletes need to give their bodies time to rest and recover after intense activity to prevent overuse injuries, we need to give our bodies time to rest and recover after more intense periods of fasting.

I just spent several chapters teaching you about how great fasting is for the body, so in the tradition of "if a little is good, then *more* must be better," we need to examine the specific reasons why this isn't always the case. Just the right amount of fasting is a great thing, but too much fasting is not.

Let's talk about how fasting affects our metabolic rates. Think back to the study I mentioned in the first chapter.[2] The subjects were monitored periodically as they fasted for seventy-two hours. Their resting metabolic rates went up by hour twelve, continued to go up through hour thirty-six, and then began to head downward by hour seventy-two. While their RMR was still higher at the seventy-two-hour mark than it had been at hour twelve, it was on a downward trend.

The fact that RMR is on a downward trend by hour seventy-two is an important clue that even with fasting, our bodies can and will slow our metabolic rates eventually when necessary to save us from starving to death. So, at what point does our metabolic rate decline to a degree where we should be concerned? The truth is that we just don't know, and I have a hunch that it's different from person to person. What's just right for *me* may be too much for *you*.

Let's talk about the concept of extended fasting. You may wonder: What is the definition of an extended fast, or EF? There is no official medical definition that I have been able to find, so I have come up with this explanation. If you're practicing time-restricted eating with a daily eating window, that is clearly not extended fasting, because you eat daily. If you're following an up-and-down-day protocol such as ADF, you're eating every day (if you have 500-calorie down days) or every other day (if doing full fasts), and an ADF protocol also wouldn't be considered as extended fasting. So, my rule of thumb is this: any fasts beyond what would be considered part of an ADF protocol venture into extended fasting territory. As an example, a 42-hour fast may seem like a lot to someone just starting out, but since it's part of an ADF protocol, it's not an EF. If your fasting is *longer* than an ADF protocol, you're in EF territory.

One proponent of extended fasting for health benefits is Dr. Joel Fuhrman, and he has worked with many patients doing therapeutic fasting to combat a whole host of health challenges. Even though he promotes the concept of medically supervised extended fasts in his book *Fasting and Eating for Health,* he admits, "Fasting slows down the metabolism, and this lowered metabolic rate can last for four to six weeks after the fast." (It is important to remember that he is discussing extended fasting here, and not intermittent fasting.)

Based on all this information, I don't recommend extended fasting for weight loss, and in practice, I have seen it backfire for many. During my years in the intermittent fasting community, I have watched all sorts of enthusiastic IFers follow the extended fasting path. Here is how it frequently plays out: They do their first extended fast, and they feel great. Not only do they feel great, but they drop several pounds quickly. This inspires them to keep pushing themselves further and further along the extended fast path. They lose lots and lots of weight quickly. Then something happens. They start to feel an increased urge to binge after a long fast. When that happens, they feel ashamed, and this leads them to believe that they must be "weak," so they vow to fast even more in response to their periods of overeating. The sad conclusion to this tale is generally rapid weight regain and a tendency to binge that doesn't seem to go away.

Why does this happen? Well, think about what we learned from studying the Minnesota Starvation Experiment in the introduction. Our bodies fight back when they feel that we are in danger. Not only do our metabolic rates fall, but we get an intense signal from our hunger hormones to EAT! EAT NOW!

Never forget this: when you are over-fasting, your body will send you a very distinct signal: the urge to binge. Never ignore this signal. It is absolutely a red flag.

If and when you want to experiment with longer fasts for the health benefits, please make sure that you are doing so safely. I would never recommend that you do a fast beyond seventy-two hours unless you are under direct medical supervision. Even fasts shorter than that can be too much for your body, so proceed with caution when exploring the world of extended fasts. And please don't repeat these longer fasts frequently. I would never recommend that anyone do a fast of seventy-two hours more frequently than once every month at the very soonest, and really, more like once a season, and only for the health benefits.

RED FLAG TWO: DISORDERED EATING BEHAVIOR

Sometimes when you tell others that you are living an intermittent fasting lifestyle, they may say, "Wow! That sounds like an eating disorder!" Sigh. That's frustrating to those of us who understand that intermittent fasting is the health plan with a side effect of weight loss.

One reason for this misconception is that fasting is a *tool* that someone with an eating disorder might abuse, leading to the mistaken idea that fasting was the problem. It's really important to understand that fasting was just the tool, while the eating disorder *itself* was the actual problem. Consider the overuse of laxatives, which are another tool that can be abused by some people who are suffering from an eating disorder. Just as using a laxative when you are constipated is not disordered behavior, fasting as a part of a healthy lifestyle is also not disordered behavior.

When professionals diagnose an eating disorder, there are certain well-defined criteria that form the basis for their diagnosis.[3] As an example, with anorexia nervosa, a diagnosis can be based on a patient's refusal to maintain a body weight within healthy parameters and/or body-perception problems where someone is actually underweight but sees themselves as overweight. With bulimia nervosa, common signs are periods of binge-eating behavior followed by any type of purging and/or excess food restriction to "make up" for the bingeing. If you see any of those signs in yourself, it's time to get help from a trained counselor or other medical professional.

Research on fasting and eating disorders is limited. In one study of ADF and disordered eating behavior, they found that an eight-week ADF protocol led to a *decrease* in binge behavior among participants, which is a good sign.[4] Also, there was no increase in any type of disordered eating behavior during those eight weeks, which is another good sign.

Never forget this: eating disorders are complex. While fasting in and of itself isn't going to cause someone to develop an eating disorder, someone with a predisposition to an eating disorder may find that fasting exacerbates the condition.

If you get to the point where you never want to eat and all you want is fasting, fasting, and more fasting, that is not a good sign. If you find yourself on the "I need to do longer and longer fasts" train, you may need to speak to a medical professional or a counselor trained in working with people with eating disorders. And be honest with yourself if you start to see danger signs. We want everyone to have great results *and* be healthy and safe.

RED FLAG THREE: PHYSICAL MATURITY

The obesity epidemic isn't just a problem with adults these days; according to the CDC (Centers for Disease Control and Prevention), the incidence of obesity among kids and teens has more than *tripled* since the 1970s.[5] With statistics like those, it can be easy to think the answer to this problem is to put our kids and teens on an intermittent fasting protocol, pronto.

Actually, no. Intermittent fasting is not recommended for bodies that are still growing and developing physically. Children and teens who are not fully mature have different nutritional needs than those of us living in adult bodies. Even in the Muslim faith, where Ramadan fasting is an important part of their religious practice, kids are usually not expected to participate until they have gone through puberty.[6]

Once your teen has gone through puberty, have a conversation with your teen's pediatrician if your teen has expressed interest in following an intermittent fasting regimen, to make sure it is appropriate for their current developmental stage.

In the meantime, what do you do if you have a child or teen who is overweight? The subject of kids and weight is a tough one. First, I think it's key to not focus on weight at all with a kid or teen. There is some evidence it does more harm than good in the long run.

One suggestion is to limit snacking (for everyone in the family, not just the family members who you feel may be overweight). Frequent snacking isn't something anyone needs to do. In terms of foods, have healthy options around the house for everyone. Serve high-quality foods at mealtimes.

And while you should never place a child or teen on an intermittent fasting protocol (unless your teen is past puberty and the pediatrician has okayed it), don't force a kid to eat when he or she is not hungry, meaning that if they naturally don't like to eat breakfast, don't force it. Instead, teach your kids to listen to their bodies and eat only when they are hungry. I know this is a lesson many of us wish we had learned as kids!

RED FLAG FOUR: PREGNANCY

Doctors who promote IF all say the same thing: they don't recommend IF for women who are pregnant. Think about this—we have learned that autophagy increases during fasting. We also know that autophagy is a process that breaks things down in our bodies and recycles them. I'm pretty sure that that is not a process we want going on when we are trying to build a healthy baby.

According to Dr. Cecily Clark-Ganheart, an ob-gyn who is a big fan of intermittent fasting in general: "We do not know enough regarding the interactions of fasting on fetal health, particularly as it applies to weight; therefore, pregnancy is not the time to experiment. Prioritize a real-foods approach, coupled with responsible weight gain, and focus on NUTRITION as the building blocks of life. Pregnancy only requires an additional 300 calories/day, the equivalent of one avocado per day."

Listen to Dr. Clark-Ganheart and save IF for later! It will be here waiting for you when you are ready.

RED FLAG FIVE: BREASTFEEDING

Just as with red flag four about women who are pregnant, doctors who promote IF all say the same thing about women who are breastfeeding: IF is not recommended.

You may think the only issue is milk supply, and as long as a mother has a sufficient supply, then all is well. Actually, it is a lot more complicated than that.

According to the book *Breastfeeding and Human Lactation,* "Fad or rapid weight loss programs should be avoided because fat-soluble environmental contaminants and toxins stored in body fat are released into the milk when caloric intake is severely restricted."[7] Since we burn stored body fat during IF, it makes sense that those toxins would be released with IF, as well.

As a mother, I wouldn't have wanted to do anything that would risk the health of my baby in any way, and I am sure that you would agree. Intermittent fasting will be there for you when your baby is fully weaned, and until then, focus on eating nourishing foods for both you *and* your baby.

In summary, here are the five fasting red flags:

RED FLAGS	WARNING SIGNS	WHAT TO DO
Red flag one: Over-fasting	Frequent use of extended fasting (beyond an ADF protocol), especially when feeling the urge to binge following fasting	Ease up on the fasting. Balance fasting and feasting until it feels right for your body.
Red flag two: Disordered eating behavior	Pressure to fast more and more and eat less and less, or a preoccupation with maintaining a weight that is lower than the recommended healthy range for your height	Check with a medical professional or an eating disorder counselor if you find that you may be showing signs of disordered eating.
Red flag three: Physical maturity	A child or teen is not yet fully developed physically	Consult with your child's pediatrician to see if your teen is sufficiently mature physically before beginning an intermittent fasting regimen.
Red flag four: Pregnancy	A positive pregnancy test	Don't begin an intermittent fasting regimen when you are pregnant, and if you have been doing IF prior to pregnancy, stop as soon as you know that you are pregnant.
Red flag five: Breastfeeding	Your child is still breastfeeding	Don't begin an intermittent fasting regimen until your baby is weaned.

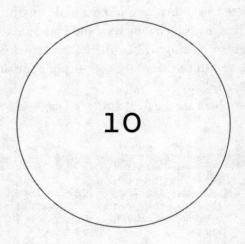

10

FAST START:
YOUR FIRST TWENTY-EIGHT DAYS

Welcome to the 28-Day FAST Start! In the FAST Start, you will:

> **F** = **Fast Clean**
>
> **A** = **Adapt**
>
> **S** = **Settle In**
>
> **T** = **Tweak**

These are the four cornerstones of the FAST Start:

1. **F= Fast Clean** This is not negotiable. Every minute you are
   fasting, follow the guidelines for the clean fast. During the
   first twenty-eight days, stick to items from the Yes column only,

and don't experiment with any of the items that are in the gray area.

2. *A= Adapt* You will ignite your fat-burning superpower, and your body will physically adapt, learning how to tap into your fat stores over time.

3. *S= Settle In* For each of the four weeks, you will settle into a predictable fasting routine. Embrace the changes that you experience along the way (even the challenging ones!), and take note of how you feel as the weeks progress.

4. *T= Tweak* While I will suggest an overall fasting routine for each week based on your personality type, feel free to change from one approach to another if you need to. Just because you decided you wanted to "rip off the Band-Aid" on day 1, that doesn't mean that you are stuck there! Head on down to the Easy Does It Approach if you need to. It's okay! You can also tweak the time of day where your eating window falls from day to day to see what feels right to you.

Think of this first twenty-eight days as the time when you will lay the foundation for your intermittent fasting practice. This will allow your body to adjust to fasting and for you to ignite your innate fat-burning superpower that you learned about in chapter 1.

Once you commit to the 28-Day FAST Start, it's important to be consistent with some sort of daily fasting time for the entire 28-day period. It's a lot harder to start and stop and start and stop, because your body never gets a chance to adapt. When that happens, you are continually doing the hard part over and over again, and you never get to the part where it becomes easier. And trust me, new IFer, it *will* get easier! If it didn't, none of us could do this long term. Once you adjust, you won't believe how great you feel, and you also won't believe that you ever used to eat all day.

But first you have to give your body a consistent beginning and have patience with yourself as your body learns to do this new thing.

It's important to know one other thing before you begin:

DO NOT EXPECT TO LOSE ANY WEIGHT OR ANY INCHES DURING THE FIRST TWENTY-EIGHT DAYS....WHAT?!?!?!

You may be saying, "But, Gin! I am doing this so I will lose weight!"

Yes. You heard me correctly. You should not expect to lose any weight or inches during the first twenty-eight days. Keep in mind that this is not like other diet plans where you are promised exciting results in the first few weeks. No, the weight will not fall right off. This FAST Start may not be easy. You may not become measurably smaller during this phase.

It's important to understand that this FAST Start is for *adjusting* to IF *only*. It is for **nailing** the clean fast and teaching your body how to access your stored body fat for fuel.

Of course, you *might* lose some pounds. You *might* lose inches or drop sizes. But you should not *expect to*. Managing your expectations is a very important step along the way. Remember those diets of the past that promised you'd lose ten pounds in a week? Remember how disappointed you were when that didn't happen?

Before I go into specifics for each of the three FAST Start options, it's time to take some baseline measurements. I promise that it is worth it, so please do *not* skip this step. You will be very glad to have this data twenty-eight days from now.

Then . . . and this might be scary . . . you are going to put away your scale, tape measure, and camera for the next twenty-eight days. I am not kidding, and this is a very important part of the process. Trust me.

On day 0, which is the day before you begin IF, carve out some time and get a notebook or an app (or write right here in the book, if you like to do that sort of thing) and record this information:

Day 0...Starting tomorrow!

Date: _____

Starting weight: _____

Measurements:

Bust or chest: _____

Waist: _____

Hips: _____

Right thigh: _____

Left thigh: _____

You can track other areas as well if you would like to. There are many places where you might want to measure yourself, so the choice is yours. If you are not sure about *how* to measure yourself accurately, do a Google search or find an instructional video on YouTube that shows you proper measuring technique.

In addition to these measurements, take photos of yourself from the front, from the side, and from the back. If possible, get someone else to take them for you . . . but mirror selfies also work. Choose an outfit that is just a little too tight right now. You will wear the same exact clothes when you take new photos in twenty-eight days.

Keep one thing in mind: the data you record on day 0 is just that. It's simply information. Don't forget that the FAST Start period is for giving your body time to adjust to the clean fast, and I want you to release all weight-loss expectations during this period.

•

Now, let's go through each of the four cornerstones of the FAST Start one by one!

F = FAST CLEAN

The most important concept of all is to nail the clean fast *first*, because that is how your body learns to access your stored fat. From day 1, the clean fast is nonnegotiable, and if you don't remember why, go back and read the clean fast chapters (chapters 4 and 5) now.

Except for the ease-in meals outlined in the Easy Does It Approach (which I will explain in a minute), I want to encourage you to follow this very important advice:

DO NOT CHANGE WHAT YOU ARE EATING YET.

Yes. It's true. I don't want you to begin intermittent fasting *and* change your diet at the same time. Never forget that this is not one of those plans that requires that you eat special foods, and in the next section of the book, you will learn why there is no one-size-fits-all way to eat (so including a meal plan in this book would actually be ridiculous). While you will most definitely fine-tune what you are eating over time (almost all of us do!), this is not yet the time.

So, when you begin IF, continue eating *the way you were most recently eating*. There are a couple of important reasons why this is the recommended approach.

1. If you try to clean up your diet while you are adjusting to IF, you are likely to become overwhelmed with too many changes at once. That is a quick trip to diet burnout. Remember that this is a process! You have plenty of time to make dietary changes along the way if you want to. Later.

2. The flip side is this: if you *have* been following a fairly "clean" diet (or another type of dietary approach such as keto, vegetarian, etc.), you may be tempted to start IF and reintroduce ALL THE THINGS at the same time. That is also a bad idea. You don't want

to shock your body in that way, so plan to gradually reintroduce foods after the 28-Day FAST Start is over if you would like to. You have plenty of time to add those foods back later, if you want to do so *and* if they are well tolerated by your body.

To clarify, if you were following the _____ diet (fill in the blank with whatever you have been doing), keep following it for now. If you have been following the keto diet, keep following it. If you have been "eating clean," keep eating clean. If you were eating the SAD (Standard American Diet), keep doing that, as well. Your *one goal* for the FAST Start is to nail the clean fast without making any other changes.

A = ADAPT

Now that you're on the eve of beginning, you're probably nervous. Can you do it? Will you be able to survive day 1? Will you be *hangry*? Let's take a minute to talk about what physical changes to expect as your body adapts to fasting.

When you begin fasting, your body is not going to know what's happening at first. Remember that your body is used to a steady supply of glucose from what you've been feeding it for breakfast, lunch, dinner, and snacks. You may know in your head that you have *plenty* of fuel stored on (and within) your body, but your brain will be searching for the easy-to-access glucose from food that it's used to. When you stop putting fuel *in* throughout the day, your body might pitch a fit at first. You may experience headaches and general tiredness or feel like you're dragging around through a pit of Jell-O. (Take some time off from your normal exercise routine if you need to; I promise that it gets so much easier to work out in the fasted state once your body adjusts to using fat for fuel. More about this in chapter 21.)

Remember that before your body can turn to your stored body

fat for fuel, you first have to deplete the stored glycogen in your liver. When you near the bottom of your stored liver glycogen, you'll probably feel even draggier than you did before! It's common for people to begin IF, have a few tough days, and then feel better for a couple of weeks, only to hit a wall around week 3 or 4. If that happens to you, understand that this is a good sign! It means you're just about to make the switch to fat burning. The process of depleting liver glycogen and flipping the metabolic switch may take a couple of weeks (or even longer!) of a consistent fasting practice. Some people don't get to this point until week 7 or 8, in fact.

How do you know that you've made the switch? There are several signs:

- All of a sudden, fasting gets easier.

- Mental clarity increases.

- You have consistent energy during the fast.

- Hunger goes down during the fast.

- You may have a telltale taste in your mouth that indicates you're in ketosis. This taste isn't perceived the same exact way by everyone, but you may notice it as metallic, salty, sweet, or like acetone nail-polish remover. If you get a different kind of taste in your mouth that coincides with the other signs from this list, it's a good indication that you're in ketosis! And what if you never get the taste in your mouth? Does that mean you are doing something wrong? No! Not everyone gets it. Don't stress about it.

We also need to address one of the most common questions that people worry about as they are beginning an intermittent fasting lifestyle: *What if I get hungry???*

For some reason, we have been trained by modern society to never ever, *ever* allow ourselves to be hungry. We are encouraged to have snacks with us at all times, in fact. I remember those days from before I was an IFer: I would sometimes eat a snack *just in case*, even when I wasn't hungry. That's how scared we are to feel a twinge of hunger! (I think the snack food companies invented this train of thought, by the way.)

Yes, you will have periods of hunger as your body adjusts to IF, and you'll even experience some degree of hunger once you *do* adjust . . . hunger comes and goes for all of us, even those of us with years of IF experience! You'll likely be surprised, however, to hear that hunger doesn't build and build until you just can't take it anymore. Actually, what happens is that you'll have a few waves of easy-to-ignore hunger that pass by quickly, particularly if you keep yourself busy. It's even more interesting to note that some of the rumbles we *think* are hunger are actually just mechanical actions of our stomachs! Until that rumble passes, take a drink of water and imagine that your body is tapping into your stored fat right at that very moment! #BurnBaby-Burn.

If you ever experience nausea, shakiness, or dizziness, go ahead and open your window. Don't try to push through that; you can fast again tomorrow! Remember that you have the rest of your life to get this right.

There is one other important feature of the adjustment period that I want to mention: the urge to overeat during your eating window. Remember what I taught you in earlier chapters: when our bodies are not well fueled, ghrelin (the hunger hormone) increases in response. When your body is still adjusting to IF, you are *not yet well fueled during the fast*. Your body is *not* accessing your fat stores efficiently, so your body responds by ramping up hunger. When your eating window opens, you may feel like a bottomless pit and like you can't get enough to eat. Don't worry—this is normal! You aren't doomed to fail, and this phase doesn't last forever (see chapter 16 for more information about this magical concept). Once your body ignites your fat-burning superpower, you'll be well fueled during the fast by your own fat, and your appetite should settle down. By the way, this overeating phase is one reason why people frequently don't lose weight (or may even gain weight) during the adjustment period, and it doesn't mean that IF isn't working for you. When you understand the physical mechanisms at play, you can relax into the process. Over time, our goal is to learn how to eat until satisfied and not stuffed, but during the FAST Start, it may be difficult to know when to stop eating . . . for now.

S = SETTLE IN

So . . . now that you understand some of the stages that you'll go through as your body adapts to IF, it's time to decide which of the three FAST Start plans is likely to be the best fit for you. Take this short quiz to figure it out. (Or you can skip the quiz and go straight to the three plans and make your own choice. I have to admit—I am a sucker for a quiz, since I am a retired teacher. If you don't want to take a quiz, I forgive you. This is one more way that we are all different.) This isn't a quiz that you can fail, which is good news.

1. **In the past, when you have started a new eating plan, which best describes you:**

   a) I like to read about the plan, spend several weeks gathering resources, and then ease my way in.

   b) I make do with the foods I already have in my kitchen and gradually implement the suggestions over time.

   c) I throw away all noncompliant foods and restock my kitchen completely to match my new plan. Let's go!

2. **Which describes your decision-making process?**

   a) I like to take my time before coming to a decision, carefully weighing out all the pros and cons. I usually make some sort of list or ask for the opinion of others before deciding. I may have trouble making the decision.

b) I think about the options carefully, and then feel confident in my decision.

c) I immediately know what my decision will be based on intuition and what feels right.

3. **What has tripped you up the most on past diet or health plans?**

a) I am easily overwhelmed when there are too many changes at once.

b) I don't always give myself enough time to adapt to the plan.

c) I am usually impatient and looking for quick results.

4. **How do you face a difficult challenge?**

a) If it seems too difficult, I may be discouraged and give up.

b) With time and effort, I usually accomplish what I set out to do.

c) Bring it on! I can do anything I set my mind to.

5. **How is your health?**

a) I have some health challenges, but my doctor said it is okay for me to start IF.

b) I am in pretty good health overall.

c) I am as healthy as a horse, thankyouverymuch.

Time to score the quiz!

Give yourself 0 points for every A, 2 points for every B, and 4 points for every C.

If you scored 0–4, you should start with the Easy Does It Approach.

If you scored a 6, you should consider either the Easy Does It or Steady Build Approach.

If you scored an 8–12, you should start with the Steady Build Approach.

If you scored a 14, you should consider either the Steady Build or the Rip Off the Band-Aid Approach.

If you scored a 16–20, you should start with the Rip Off the Band-Aid Approach.

Feel free to ignore this quiz if you find it hokey, and choose whatever plan feels right to *you*. Remember—*you* are in charge at all times.

•

Note: You may remember from the eating window chapter that there is no "best" time to have your eating window. Still, based on the informal survey of intermittent fasters, I found that 61 percent of IFers in my online community prefer an evening window while 25 percent prefer a midday eating window. For that reason, the FAST Start plan has been designed with an early evening eating window as the goal. Feel free to adjust the window timing on any of these approaches as it feels right to you.

Now, let's dig into the three FAST Start approaches and see just how to implement each of them. Even though there are many tools in your intermittent fasting toolbox, the FAST Start will focus on the eating-window approach to IF. After the first twenty-eight days are over, you will be free to pull out other tools as you see fit and experiment with the other approaches.

THE EASY DOES IT APPROACH		
Days 1–7	12-hour window	Low-carb ease-in breakfast, low-carb ease-in lunch, regular dinner
Days 8–14	10-hour window	Late low-carb ease-in breakfast *or* early low-carb ease-in lunch, low-carb ease-in snack, regular dinner
Days 15–21	8-hour window	Low-carb ease-in lunch, regular dinner
Days 22–28	6-hour window	Low-carb ease-in lunch *or* low-carb ease-in snack, regular dinner

In this approach, you're starting out in week 1 with three meals a day in a twelve-hour eating window. Notice that this plan includes some low-carb "ease-in" meals that will help your body lower insulin levels (our bodies release less insulin in response to lower-carb meals) while still eating three times a day at first. Have a low-carb breakfast and a low-carb lunch, and then eat the type of dinner that you're used to (dinner doesn't need to be low-carb unless you have already been living a low-carb lifestyle; remember that other than these low-carb ease-in meals, we aren't changing *what* we eat during the FAST Start, only *when* we eat).

Each week, you tighten up your eating window by a couple of hours, until you finally end up with a window of about six hours containing either two meals or a snack and a meal.

THE STEADY BUILD APPROACH		
Days 1–7	8-hour window	Lunch, dinner
Days 8–14	7-hour window	Lunch, dinner
Days 15–21	6-hour window	Lunch *or* snack, dinner
Days 22–28	5-hour window	Snack, dinner

In this approach, you start off skipping breakfast on day 1, and BOOM! You're doing it! Stick to clean-fast-approved beverages all morning, and eat your typical lunch followed by your typical dinner within an eight-hour eating window.

Each week, you shorten your eating window by an hour, and you end up in week 4 with an eating window of five hours that contains a snack and a meal.

THE RIP OFF THE BAND-AID APPROACH		
Days 1–7	6-hour window	Lunch, dinner
Days 8–14	6-hour window	Lunch *or* snack, dinner
Days 15–21	5-hour window	Lunch *or* snack, dinner
Days 22–28	4-hour window	Snack, dinner

In this approach, you are maximizing your fasting time starting on day 1, with a six-hour window and therefore eighteen hours of daily fasting. The first week you skip breakfast and eat two meals, and over the course of weeks 2 and 3, you can choose to either eat lunch or transition lunch into more of a snack. In week 4, you end up with an eating window of four hours that contains a snack and a meal.

You may still have one nagging question after reading these plans: *What's the difference between a snack and a meal???*

Believe it or not, I've seen that question a lot. I want to encourage you to not get too hung up on terminology, but to decide if something qualifies as a meal, I ask myself this: If a friend invited me over for dinner and served this to me, would I consider it to have been an actual dinner? If not, it's probably a snack. Go with your gut here. However, since our goal every day is to eat until we are satisfied and not stuffed, it doesn't matter what you call it, now does it?

T = TWEAK

At any point, remember that you can move from one plan to another if you need to. Started off too aggressively? Drop back to a gentler approach. Finding the plan to be almost *too* easy? Go up a level to a more aggressive approach. *You* are in control the whole time.

In each of these plans, I suggested an eating window that emphasizes dinner as the main meal of the day, since that is the way most of the intermittent fasters in my community structure their days. Never forget, however, that *you* are in charge here, not me. If you would rather eat breakfast and lunch and skip dinner, go for it! That might be *your* perfect plan.

After following the FAST Start for twenty-eight days, it's time to repeat your measurements and photos:

Day 29 . . . FAST Start completed!

Date: _____

Current weight: _____

Measurements:

Bust or chest: _____

Waist: _____

Hips: _____

Right thigh: _____

Left thigh: _____

Put on the same outfit that you wore on day 0 and take photos from the same exact angles that you did before: front, side, and back. Try to re-create the photos as closely as possible. Compare the photos from day 0 to the ones you took on day 29.

Here is something that is *really important* that I've already mentioned: You may not have lost a single pound. Your measurements may not have changed at all. Your photos may look exactly the same. Or your weight and/or measurements might be *up*. Your clothes might be *tighter*.

Deep breath. That is okay. It's *all* okay. The 28-Day FAST Start is *not* the weight-loss phase; it's the adjustment phase. Now that your body has had twenty-eight days to adjust to IF, you are ready to begin weighing daily, as explained in chapter 18. You will begin taking biweekly measurements and progress photos now. The FAST Start is over, and *now* is the time to expect slow-yet-steady progress. See chapter 18 for an in-depth discussion of all the ways you may want to track your progress, and how to know that you're getting the results you are hoping for.

Anyway, CONGRATULATIONS to you! Now that you've completed the FAST Start, you're ready to learn how to "tweak it till it's easy!"

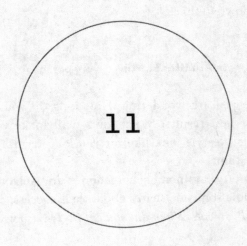

11

TWEAK IT TILL IT'S EASY

You made it! You have finished the FAST Start, and now you are ready to take charge of your own IF plan going forward!

Ready, set, go!

Um. What now? WHAT DO I DO, GIN???

Great question! You may be used to flipping through the pages of any new diet book looking for the exact "diet" or "meal plan" that the author has laid out for you. You know, the weekly schedule that everyone needs to follow to find success. Usually, there are phases and recipes and grocery lists and step-by-step guidelines for every part of the process. Well, you won't find that here.

IF is not a diet, and there is no one-size-fits-all plan. This may be scary, because you are used to someone else telling you exactly what to do. I am not going to do that for you. As I told you in the beginning pages of this book, *you* are in charge. Why? Because I want *you* to feel empowered to find the right IF routine that works for you. It won't look exactly like mine.

It comes down to this:

Intermittent fasting is *very* personal.

I am sure you are wondering: How long do you need to fast every day for best results? What foods will make you feel best? What will the lifestyle look like for *you* long term? These are all excellent questions!

There's a pretty common phenomenon in any weight-loss support group. Any time someone shares about their success, others always ask: *What did you eat? When did you eat it? Tell us exactly what you did!*

It's natural for us to think there is a magical answer out there that is the same for everyone. After all, isn't that what every diet plan has *always* told us? Do *x, y,* and *z,* exactly like this, and you'll lose weight.

How did that work for you? It probably *didn't* work for you long term, in fact, or you wouldn't be here.

Remember these three simple words: FAST. FEAST. REPEAT.

Your intermittent fasting lifestyle will have periods of fasting, periods of feasting, and you will repeat, alternating fasting with feasting. That's it.

And also remember this: ONE SIZE DOES NOT FIT ALL!

This brings up a very important point, and the point of this chapter. We have one more saying in our community that is the key to your personal success:

Tweak it till it's easy.

That saying is meant to empower you. After the 28-Day FAST Start, your body is getting into the fasting groove. While I did give you a few schedules to choose from and follow as your body adjusted to intermittent fasting and fat burning, your next step is to experiment with the various tools from the fasting toolbox.

We are taking off the training wheels, and you are ready to ride the bike! And like a kid riding for the first time, you may worry that you can't do it without me holding on to the back of the bike.

You can! I promise you can.

Imagine me running along beside you, encouraging you every inch of the way as you begin experimenting with the tools from your IF toolbox. You might fall down, but you'll dust yourself off and get right back on the bike!

As you experiment, remember that other than the clean fast (which is NOT optional, I promise), don't try to fit what you are doing into someone else's recommendations of how and when to fast (or even what you should be eating). Listen to how you feel over time and live your life as a study of one. The one that you are studying is *you*, and no one else knows what feels right to you better than, well, *you*.

The intermittent fasting lifestyle that makes *me* feel best is not necessarily the one that will make *you* feel best. And guess what else? The fasting pattern that feels effortless to you today may not feel effortless to you next month. You may need to go back to the toolbox, pick a new strategy, and try a different fasting pattern for a while. Don't be afraid to mix and match!

Tweak it till it's easy!

And if you need to, tweak it again. And again. And again. This is a lifestyle, and you have the rest of your life to get it right. (And sometimes, you won't get it right. That is okay, too.)

How do you know if something is working? Well, as I've already taught you, your body has amazing feedback mechanisms built in that are meant to keep you alive. If you feel better and better over time, and your fasting pattern feels easy and natural, that is a really good sign that your body is content and what you are doing is working well for you.

How do you know if something is *not* working? Again, you can rely on your body's feedback. If you feel worse and worse over time, and it begins to feel harder and harder to fast, or you feel the urge to binge and that urge is getting worse, that is a really bad sign that your body is distressed by what you are doing, and something is *not* working well for you. Perhaps you need to take a gentler approach to fasting for a time.

It's perfectly fine to cycle through a gentler approach (such as 16:8) for a while and then spend a short time trying something more aggressive like 22:2. Alternate. Pick and choose. Try out different tools, cycle through approaches, and try things on for size to see if they fit.

As you tweak, there is something very important to keep in mind: give each tweak enough time. When you switch something up, make sure you give it a chance so you can see how your body adapts. One example may be trying an up-and-down-day protocol. Don't expect to do one down day and then know how it works for you based on that short time. You may need to try it for a couple of weeks (or a month!) to see how your body adapts and to see if it begins to feel natural.

I really want to reiterate this concept, because it's so important: **After every tweak, give it some time to see how it's working for you.**

You may still wonder, though: What do I mean by "working"?

To determine if a tweak is working for you, consider these questions:

- How do you feel *emotionally*? This one is important! We *always* want to be in a good place mentally.

    Here's an example: if you try an ADF protocol for a month and you dread every single down day, and you feel like you want to binge throughout every single up day, then you know that this isn't working well for you emotionally.

Don't forget, though—make sure that you give it a few weeks to see if you adjust. A new routine may be hard for the first two weeks and then suddenly you're in the groove and you love it. Tweak it till it's easy!

- How do you feel *physically*? We have learned that it can take the body time to adapt to a new routine, so expect some sort of adjustment phase when you make a change in your fasting schedule. After giving your body time to adjust, see how you feel. It's always a good sign to find that you have great energy and mental clarity during the fast. If you start to feel worse and worse physically after a few weeks, that is a sign that you need to make a different tweak. Tweak it till it's easy!

- Are you getting the *results* you were hoping for? Remember that weight loss is not the only metric we consider here. As I've already taught you, IF is the health plan with a side effect of weight loss, so pay attention to every single improvement! If you aren't losing weight but you feel ten years younger and pesky ailments are vanishing, you *are* getting some amazing results, no matter what the scale or tape measure says!

  Also, make sure you are measuring progress in several ways. At the beginning and end of the FAST Start, you weighed, you took photos, and you took measurements. Use all these tools to see if your body is changing. (More about this in chapter 18.) If weeks go by with no changes at all, you know it may be time for a tweak. Tweak it till it's easy!

If you feel good emotionally and physically and you are seeing some sort of measurable results, then you know that whatever you are doing is working for you!

All right, then! Now that you understand how to tweak it till it's easy, it's time to talk about the feast!

PART II

FEAST.

After you've settled into your intermittent fasting lifestyle (and *after* the twenty-eight days of the FAST Start are over), you may be ready to focus on *what* or *how much* you are eating. Part 2 of *Fast. Feast. Repeat.* answers some of your most common questions: *What the heck should I EAT? Should I count calories? Track fat grams? Limit carbs? Does food quality matter? Are there foods that should be avoided? Can I really eat ANYTHING I WANT? Help!*

Don't worry! I will teach you how to become an intuitive intermittent faster by learning to recognize the natural cues that your body sends you. Over time, you'll learn to once again trust in yourself and your ability to choose healthy (and delicious!) foods that work well for your unique body . . . while still enjoying delicious treats! When you are eating nutritious foods that satisfy your body and fill you up *and* allowing yourself to also add in the treats you love, every day really does feel like something to celebrate . . . a feast!

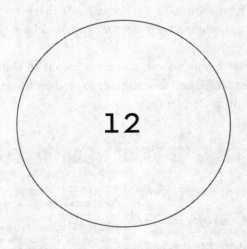

12

"DELAY, DON'T DENY"

My first book was called *Delay, Don't Deny,* and this phrase has become a mantra for many of us in the IF community. By fasting clean, we *delay* our eating until our eating window or our up day, and we *don't deny* ourselves of the foods we want to eat! Now that you are living the Delay, Don't Deny intermittent fasting lifestyle along with hundreds of thousands of other DDDers, let's take some time to understand the *food* part of the equation. It can be the most difficult piece of the puzzle for many.

Our goal is to learn to listen to our bodies over time, choose delicious and nutritious foods that support vibrant health, and also save some room in our lives for our favorite treats. This is certainly different from diets of the past where you had to deny yourself of everything that you wanted to eat.

When you eat satisfying meals full of high-quality foods and also enjoy your favorite treats, every day truly feels like a celebratory feast!

In the coming chapters of the Feast section of the book, we are going to talk a lot about how to choose foods that work well for your body. *Food quality absolutely does matter,* and I am going to teach you why that is true.

Before we talk about food, however, I want to show you a very important graphic. Take a few minutes to read each section carefully. Study the wording. Ponder these concepts.

DELAY, DON'T DENY (DDD) INTERMITTENT FASTING	
DDD is a lifestyle.	DDD is not a diet.
DDD is the health plan with a side effect of weight loss.	DDD is NOT a "lose weight quickly!" or "drop sizes in days!" approach.
DDD is FREEDOM from counting calories, points, or macros. YOU are in charge of figuring out what works for you. Remember one thing: you have the rest of your life to get this right!	DDD is NOT a prescriptive approach or one-size-fits-all. Everyone tweaks to find their own unique approach, which takes time.
DDD is a way to connect with your satiety signals and stop eating when you have had enough.	DDD is NOT permission to eat more food than you need just because you "can," or your window is still open.

Throughout both the Feast and the Repeat sections of this book, we will be exploring all the concepts from this graphic (and more) in greater detail. But first, let's unpack the most important phrase of the DDD lifestyle: **DELAY, DON'T DENY!**

Many people are excited about a DDD lifestyle because of the promise of enjoying all the foods we have worried about and restricted for so long. We have "permission" to eat foods we love again.

Sometimes, that leads to overindulgence, as we gleefully add back all these various foods. This can lead to weight stability rather than weight loss, or even weight GAIN, if you are coming out of a restrictive diet.

The phrase *Delay, Don't Deny* becomes our mantra. How can we think about it in a new way?

The word *delay* is easy to understand. We delay until our eating window (or up day). Easy-peasy.

The phrase *don't deny* is a little more nuanced, however. The way you interpret it can be the difference between success and failure for you.

Don't deny means that there are no foods to avoid. There are no lists of "good foods" and "bad foods." You are in charge of what you are eating at all times, and you really don't have to give up your favorite foods. Even when I teach you about why it is important to choose highly nutritious foods in chapter 17, that doesn't mean that you also have to shun delicious treats forever. (Though you'll probably be amazed by how your definition of "delicious" changes over time . . . IF eventually turns most of us into food snobs, and something you think is a delicious treat *today* may be something you turn your nose up at in the future. It happens to almost all of us as we become more in tune with our bodies. Even our tastes change. It's part of the IF magic! Food must be "window-worthy" or we don't want to waste our time with it.) While those types of foods shouldn't form the centerpiece of your overall diet, there is still room for the treats you love. Don't deny!

BUT! Understand this. *Don't deny* is not code for *eat as much food as you want without restriction because you fasted all day and now you deserve it!* Let's unpack this concept.

With *Delay, Don't Deny,* you can truly **eat whatever YOU want**!

However! That is not the same thing as *EAT WHATEVER YOU WANT!*

Confused? I get it. I just wrote the exact same words and told you that they mean different things. The key is the emphasis.

Yes. You can **eat whatever YOU want**. Notice the emphasis on the word *you*. All the foods that are on the No lists of diets you have tried in the past? If you want to eat those foods, you now have permission to eat them. You do not need to *deny* your favorite foods for the rest of your life.

No. You can't *EAT WHATEVER YOU WANT!* Sometimes, intermittent fasting is sold as "this is the plan that allows you to eat without restriction, and you can magically lose weight even while stuffing yourself with formerly forbidden foods!"

That is not true.

Remember your goals. If you are hoping to lose weight with intermittent fasting, you must tap into stored fat during the fast. You must therefore deplete your glycogen stores sufficiently to get into fat burning during the fast. If you overeat during your eating window, not only will you refill your glycogen stores, but you'll also store some of the excess food you eat as fat. You won't lose weight and you may even gain weight.

While intermittent fasting does come with some degree of hormonal and metabolic magic, it's *not* so magical that you can overeat within your eating window and still expect to lose weight.

Also, ***EAT WHATEVER YOU WANT!*** always sounds to me like the way a college freshman approaches the cafeteria during that first semester. Mom is not there telling you what to eat, so you tend to go a little nuts. (I did that. Freshman 15, anyone?)

How do we *Delay, Don't Deny* in practice?

DON'T DENY DOES MEAN:	DON'T DENY DOES NOT MEAN:
Craving tacos? *Delay, Don't Deny!* Decide to make tacos for dinner.	When your window opens, go through a drive-through and get a family-sized taco meal and eat the whole thing by yourself.
Does the pizza your coworker is eating look really good? *Delay, Don't Deny!* You can have pizza later, in your eating window . . . if you still want pizza then. Eat pizza until you are satisfied and then stop.	When it is time to eat, eat as much pizza as you can until you are stuffed and miserable.
Doughnuts in the break room? *Delay, Don't Deny!* Grab a doughnut to take home and have it later, after dinner.	Get a dozen doughnuts and eat them all to close your window.
Do you love Doritos? *Delay, Don't Deny!* Have a few Doritos as a part of your snack to open your window, along with something containing nutrients.	Open your window with a whole super-sized bag of Doritos.
Is ice cream your favorite treat? *Delay, Don't Deny!* Buy your favorite ice cream and have a small scoop to close your window.	Eat an entire container of ice cream.

So, as you see, every day, we *delay* eating, and then we *don't deny*. But we also don't have permission to overeat just because our window is open. I'll explain more about how to know when you have had enough food in chapter 16. Learning to trust your hunger and satiety signals is an important part of the process.

Besides delaying food until your eating window (or up day), you can also think of *Delay, Don't Deny* as a longer-term strategy. You may not be able to eat every single thing you want every day along the way and still lose weight. Sometimes, when the goal is weight loss, it's important to *delay* certain foods that don't align with your current goals for a little longer.

I used this *delay* strategy in 2015 as I was approaching my initial goal weight. I wanted to do something that would speed up my results . . . spring was in the air, and I needed a whole new wardrobe . . . and I wanted to be in my goal body so I could buy clothes that would fit me for more than just a few weeks. (Get used to this problem, by the way! You'll buy a new wardrobe and then shrink out of it before you know it and need to shop again. It's a pretty fabulous problem to have! Become familiar with the best secondhand and consignment shops in your town as you're losing weight—those stores will be your best friends!)

Since my goal was weight loss, I decided to *delay* both alcohol and highly processed foods for a time. I didn't give up carbs or fat, I didn't count calories, and I didn't restrict the amount of food I was eating. Instead, every day, I selected high-quality foods that made me feel full and satisfied. I literally feasted every single night, and it didn't feel at all like I was on some kind of sad diet. A typical dinner was a huge baked potato with butter and sour cream, vegetables sautéed in butter, and some fresh berries with heavy cream for dessert. Or maybe dinner would be beans and brown rice with cheese and sour cream, a huge salad, and an apple with peanut butter for dessert.

It worked! The weight melted away at the rate of about two pounds per week. Keep in mind that I had already lost about fifty-five pounds by that point, so losing the final twenty pounds in about ten weeks was a really quick rate of weight loss. The magical combination of delaying alcohol and processed foods worked amazingly well for my body. On March 15, 2015, I got on the scale and saw my goal weight flashing up at me: 135 pounds. Let the shopping begin!

"But, Gin. You told me I wasn't going to have to DENY. This sounds a lot like DENY to me."

I know, and I get it. Living inside of most of us is what I like to call our *inner toddler:* "I want it, and I want it NOW!" I *love* having a glass of wine with dinner. I also love the freedom to eat whatever I want with no restrictions. Even so, I made a conscious decision to ignore my inner toddler *for a time* and eat like a grown-up. Even though I eat what most people would call a healthy diet *now,* I ate a lot of processed foods for most of my adult life, and shifting away from those was a big change for my body. The good news is that my body loved that little shift. And so did my taste buds.

It's important to keep in mind that I didn't eat diet foods or count calories or macros. I was not *dieting* in any sense of the word. Instead, I simply delayed a few things that I knew were working against me (alcohol and overly processed foods, including sugar) and I filled up on foods that were highly nutritious and also extremely satisfying. It's also important to understand that the foods that worked very well for me—the potatoes with butter and sour cream, beans with cheese and sour cream, and so on—may *not* be foods that work well for *your* body. More about this concept in chapter 14!

Once I reached my goal weight, I added back in all the things I temporarily delayed. What I did *not* do was stop fasting! I continued living an intermittent fasting lifestyle, and my body went on to s-l-o-w-l-y lose about five more pounds over the next couple of years, without me needing to do any more delaying. It's true! I was a size 4 when I hit my goal weight in 2015. By the end of 2016, I was down another five pounds (bringing my total loss to about eighty pounds) and wearing a size 0–2. It didn't happen quickly, but my body continued to get leaner thanks to a consistent intermittent fasting practice.

Delay, Don't Deny!

Every day, you will *delay* eating until your eating window opens (or your up day begins, if you are an up-and-down-day IFer). Occasionally, you may also decide to *delay* certain foods (or alcohol) that you know are keeping you from reaching your goals. The beauty of the DDD IF lifestyle is that you don't have to delay your favorite foods forever! You genuinely won't have to spend the rest of your life denying yourself of any food that you love. Over time, you'll figure out just the right balance of **delay**ing and **don't deny**ing that will help you achieve and maintain your goal weight forever. It's such a freeing way to live! Tonight, I shall eat pizza and drink wine and tomorrow my skinny clothes will all still fit.

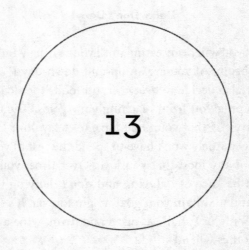

13

"DIET BRAIN"
AND HOW TO AVOID IT

Even though you are learning how to *delay* rather than *deny*, it's still important to make sure that you are choosing foods that support your body nutritionally. But what foods *should* you choose?

If you want to be really confused, go to the diet aisle of any bookstore and start reading the books on the shelves. Should we eat like cavemen? Is keto the answer for everyone? Or is it better to be vegetarian or to go full-on vegan? On the other hand, are plants paradoxically trying to kill you?

Every diet book out there promises to reveal the #OneTrueWay that we should all be eating. (One time, on a road trip, I played a game where I asked my husband to name foods, and to win I had to give the name of a diet book or protocol that had that food on the list of "forbidden" items. Yep. I could do it . . . for ANY FOOD. If you have read as many diet books as I have read in my life, you may also be able to win at this game, just as I did that day. Spoiler alert: the prize is actually total confusion and a bad case of "diet brain." The best way to "win" is to avoid playing.)

So, what is *diet brain*? It's when you no longer feel confident in making *any* food choices because of all the conflicting information out there. To illustrate the concept, these are things we have been told by various experts based on "science":

Eggs will kill you because eating them will give you high cholesterol.	*Or maybe . . .*	Eggs are one of the healthiest foods you can eat because they contain essential vitamins and nutrients, including vitamin D and choline, just to name two.
Vegetarians live longer because of all the nutrients in vegetables, and meat will rot in your intestines, which is just gross when you think about it.	*Or maybe . . .*	Most plant foods are full of antinutrients that are making you sick and you don't even know it, so avoid many if not most plant foods and eat mostly meat like the cavemen did.
Saturated fat is the worst thing you can consume, because it increases your risk of heart disease and stroke.	*Or maybe . . .*	Try a diet that is mostly fat to lose weight, and oh . . . it also LOWERS your risk of stroke.[1]
Whole grains keep you slim, so include them at every meal.	*Or maybe . . .*	Whole grains are the reason we are so fat, and they are destroying your gut, so avoid them completely.
A high-protein diet will cause you to lose fat and also help you build muscle, so eat more protein.	*Or maybe . . .*	Eating less protein is linked to longevity, so eat less protein.[2]

No wonder we are all so confused. Each one of the statements above is based on someone's analysis of nutritional studies, and here's what is even more confusing: most of those statements have a nugget of truth to them, even if they are contradictory.

Based on these confusing nutritional recommendations, we have been bombarded with news articles that scream sensational headlines at us. When you read articles with these sensational headlines, such as EATING _____ WILL CAUSE YOU TO HAVE HEART ATTACKS, YOUR DOG WILL BE MORE LIKELY TO BITE YOU, AND THE APOCALYPSE WILL BE IMMINENT (I exaggerated for emphasis, but not by much), you may be scared by them. Yes, confusing dietary advice has been plaguing us for decades now.

Deep breath, people. Taking our medical advice from headlines based on faulty studies or misinterpretation of data is what got us *into* this mess. And we have the tools to escape the madness.

Beyond the articles with their scary headlines, I would bet that we have all read multiple diet books that profess to have all the answers within their pages. Each book is *the* ideal plan, contains all the "true" science, and will solve all your health and weight problems. Most of these are written by doctors.

When you read a diet book written by a doctor, it is going to be very compelling and believable. He or she cites studies that back up every claim. As I mentioned earlier, we authors are great at cherry-picking the studies that support our own dietary beliefs, and some-times the research studies we cite within our books don't actually say what we claim they say. So, always draw your own conclusions based on the actual research studies, rather than the author's interpretation of them. (Also apply this advice to anything *I* share with you. While I pledge to never misrepresent a study on purpose, I want you to go to the source just to make sure or to gain a deeper understanding for yourself.)

Diet books all claim that their plans will help you lose weight, avoid disease, and also live longer. (As does the one you are hold-ing in your hand right now!) They have compelling stories, and each book has testimonials from people who have adopted the specific plan and reversed all their prior health conditions. (Also true for this one!) The problem is when they claim that there is a one-size-fits-all way to go about it and when they assume that all our bodies are the same, and that every person who tries their plan will be successful with it because it speaks universal truth that applies to all bodies. (And *that* is what is different about *Fast. Feast. Repeat. You* are going to design your own fasting protocol, and *you* are going to choose what foods you want to eat, because there is no such thing as a one-size-fits-all plan.)

As an example, certain books promote a low-fat lifestyle as the most health-promoting way to live. An early book is *The T-Factor Diet* by Dr. Martin Katahn. Another is *The Starch Solution* by Dr. John McDougall. These authors provide many scientific claims backed up by scientific studies. By the time you finish reading either of these books, you will be convinced that a plant-based diet high in starches and whole grains and low in fat is the best thing you can do for your health.

Then you read a book like *Grain Brain* by Dr. David Perlmutter or *Wheat Belly* by Dr. William Davis. These books tell you that the other doctors have it all wrong. Rather than eating grains, we should, in fact, *avoid* grains. These books also have scientific claims backed up by multiple scientific studies. When you read these books, you will become convinced that grains are one of the worst foods you could eat, particularly modern grains.

There are also books such as *The Art and Science of Low Carbohydrate Living* by Stephen Phinney and Jeff Volek or *The Real Meal Revolution* by Tim Noakes, Jonno Proudfoot, and Sally-Ann Creed, both of which promote exclusion of carbohydrates in favor of a higher-fat lifestyle. These books are equally as compelling and will convince you that humans should not eat starches or grains at all and that they are at the root of all our modern diseases. Scientific claims and scientific studies? Yep. All in there.

Please understand one important thing: I am not criticizing any of these authors, and I am also not claiming that their work is without merit. I wholeheartedly believe that what they write is based on a foundation of solid scientific principles and that their plans are exactly the right approach . . . for some people. Some people may thrive on a lower-fat approach, and they will feel awful and gain weight if they eat too much fat. Others may reverse many health conditions following a low-carb/high-fat approach, and there are many reasons why this is true for their bodies. (Okay, so perhaps I have just made both the low-carb community AND the low-fat community angry, but hang with me here.) Because of what we are beginning to understand about the individual differences in how our bodies work, we can say with confidence that what works for one person may not work for another.

So, why is diet brain so dangerous? By relying on diet programs and "experts" to tell us exactly *what* and *how much* to eat, we have lost the ability to trust ourselves and our bodies to guide us to the foods that work well for us. I think of my grandmother. One time she said, "I like broccoli, but it doesn't agree with me." (That may actually have been code for "I don't like broccoli, so I am going to tell you it doesn't agree with me." We will never know, but I will assume that she was telling the truth there.) Broccoli didn't work well for her body, and she could tell, so she didn't eat it. She didn't need to find a nutritional study about the dangers of broccoli or read a diet book that cautioned her to be wary of broccoli. She simply didn't eat it.

Have you ever choked down a food you don't like because a diet book told you it was a superfood? Or on the flip side, have you ever avoided a food that you *love* because you had the idea it was a "bad" food?

It's time for us to all take back the power and learn to listen to our bodies.

Let me give you an example: the humble potato. As with every food, you can get so many conflicting opinions about potatoes. Are they good for us or bad for us? Should we eat potatoes, or should we avoid them forever? Superfood or dietary demon?

One time, I heard someone say that you shouldn't eat potatoes because "they are pure sugar and when you eat one, it is *exactly* like eating spoonfuls of sugar." That's pretty alarming, isn't it? Can you imagine sitting down with a potato-sized bowl of sugar and eating it, one spoonful after another? It sounds horrifying, and who would do that??? Most of all, though, is that statement true?

Let's look at it from a nutritional perspective. Potatoes are an excellent source of vitamin C, providing as much as 30 percent of your recommended daily allowance. They contain more potassium than a banana. If you eat the skin, one potato provides about 7 percent of your daily fiber intake, which can help you feel full longer. A potato also includes about 10 percent of your daily vitamin B6 needs and 6 percent of your daily iron needs. Sugar, on the other hand, has zero nutrients (that's what they mean when they say "empty calories"). So, is a potato exactly like sugar? Nutritionally, not even close.

Since potatoes are full of nutrients, should *you* eat potatoes? Maybe the answer is *yes*, as it is for me. Maybe the answer is *no* for your body.

Once I understood how to really tune in to my body's signals, I have been able to reject diet brain forever, and this applies to potatoes. When I eat potatoes, particularly if I load them down with a hearty scoop of both butter and sour cream, I feel full and satisfied for hours. (Fun fact: during the period when I was losing weight the quickest back in 2015, losing at the rate of about two pounds per week [which is well above the typical one-pound per week average!], I ate huge baked potatoes with butter and sour cream several nights per week. They work very well for my body, even though the low-carb books would tell me that I shouldn't eat potatoes and the low-fat books would tell me that I shouldn't eat butter or sour cream and the food-combining books would tell me that it is impossible to lose weight while combining carbs and fats in one meal. Nobody told that to my body, though. My body thrives on potatoes with butter and sour cream. Could it be my Irish heritage?)

While I still read nutritional studies with interest, I don't assume that every person's body is the same, and I don't feel the need to change what I am eating to avoid (or include) certain foods based on what I read. I have taken back my power and rejected diet brain forever. Once again, food is just food, and I no longer face the thought of "eating food" with the idea that it is complicated in any way.

While it is true that some foods will work well for your body and some won't, it's *not* true that the answer is found in the pages of a prescriptive diet book.

For a more peaceful and empowered life, in fact, I would like to have you promise me that you will stop reading diet books once and for all. Clear your mind from the confusion of conflicting theories, and when you see an alarming headline du jour, you will have the power to IGNORE IT.

So? Are you ready to say goodbye to diet brain forever and take back your power once and for all? Let's learn about food!

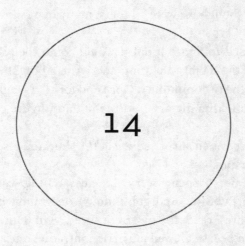

14

BIO-INDIVIDUALITY

It's true! There is NO one-size-fits-all diet plan that works for each of us. Your friend may have had amazing results following the latest high-fat keto diet plan, but when you tried it, you felt worse and worse over time . . . and you *gained* weight! In fact, you felt your best (and were your leanest!) when you followed the low-fat diets from the '90s. Is there science that explains why this might be true? I'm glad you asked! Once you learn what I am going to share with you here in this chapter, you will be cured of diet brain forever. The answer lies in the concept of bio-individuality.

When I sat down to write my second book, *Feast Without Fear,* in 2017, I had been living an intermittent fasting lifestyle for over three years, and I had been at my goal weight for over two years. I felt like I had it all figured out when it came to weight loss and weight maintenance; IF was the answer. Still, though, there was a reoccurring problem within our online IF support community; members could *not* agree on how we should all be eating.

Yep. Even though we were all IFers, many of us were still plagued by diet brain.

So, I decided to figure it out. I would comb the scientific literature, read all the dietary theories, and write a book to share what I learned with the IF community. Once and for all, I would make sense of all the conflicting dietary information and figure out the "best" way to eat.

What I discovered surprised me at the time and also cured me of my diet brain for good.

That summer, I spent every day researching: reading books, searching on PubMed, and going down one rabbit hole after another. The more I read, the more confused I got. How could scientific studies in peer-reviewed journals contradict one another? How could one renowned medical doctor write a book that said the exact opposite of another equally renowned medical doctor? My head was spinning with so much information, and I felt no closer to the answer. One day, though, I stumbled across a video that changed everything.

In a 2016 video, Dr. Eran Segal presented his scientific research in a TED Talk called "What is the Best Diet for Humans?"[1] On that day in 2017, I watched the video with my jaw on the floor. Then I watched it again. Then I made my husband watch it.

In this video, Dr. Segal presented scientific research that conclusively demonstrates that individuals have bodies that have *different responses* to the *same exact foods*.

Let me explain. Have you ever heard of the glycemic index? I'm sure you have. The glycemic index (GI) is a ranking of foods from 0 to 100, based on how much they raise our blood sugar levels. A higher GI means that the food raises your blood sugar more quickly, which results in a more rapid decline after eating. Picture your blood sugar curve as an intense roller coaster with a big climb and then you go down a huge and scary hill. We want to *avoid* that type of huge spike and rapid drop, as it's associated with negative health outcomes. Now, picture a kids' beginner roller coaster that you might put your toddler onto. It's probably got cute little caterpillar cars that you ride in, and you travel up and down a very gentle course. Gentle ups, and gentle downs. *That* is what we want from our blood glucose: lower highs and higher lows. Foods that have a lower GI lead to a smaller fluctuation in blood glucose, just like the kiddie roller coaster. The lesson from this analogy is this: for good health, avoid the scary and intense blood-sugar roller coaster (peaks followed by crashes) and stick to the cute and gentle blood-sugar caterpillar ride (slow and steady ups and downs). Having a high glucose response to your meals is a risk factor for obesity, diabetes, cardiovascular disease, and other metabolic disorders, and it's also a predictor of higher overall mortality.[2]

So, we should be very interested in determining how our bodies respond to different foods, and the glycemic index seems like it would be very helpful in that regard, which is how it was designed to be used. The glycemic index was calculated by giving a standard portion of each food to ten or more subjects, measuring their response, and then comparing that value to how they responded to pure glucose. When the two numbers are taken as a ratio, you have the glycemic index for that food. Scientists then took the results from those ten or so subjects and found the average, and then the food's glycemic index value was determined.[3]

Whenever we see the glycemic index mentioned, the number is given to us as an absolute: the glycemic index of glucose is 100. White bread is 75. Corn is 52, and ice cream is 51.[4] This concept would indicate that everyone would be better off avoiding bread and that both corn and ice cream would have a similar response for everyone, since they are very close in GI numbers.

Except that's not true.

You see, it turns out we have a *highly individual* blood glucose response to foods.

In a fascinating study, Dr. Segal and his colleagues measured the blood glucose response to a variety of meals of hundreds of participants and found that for every single food they tested, some people had a low blood glucose response, some people had a high blood glucose response, and others had a medium response. For *every food.*

This means that even though corn and ice cream have a similar glycemic index score, some subjects had a high blood glucose spike from corn and others had a low blood glucose spike from corn, and the same is true for ice cream.

Upon further analysis, they were able to use individual data from the hundreds of subjects in the test group and develop an algorithm that would predict a person's response to meals with a high level of accuracy. They found that the most important personal factors had to do with the composition of each person's gut microbiome. Yep! It's true. A person's glycemic response to foods was highly linked to the population of the little bugs that live in our intestines!

To see if this algorithm worked, they took a new group of participants and used the algorithm to predict a "good" and a "bad" diet for each of them. People followed each diet for one week without knowing which diet was which, and their blood glucose responses were tracked for the entire week.

Results were fascinating. When participants followed the diet that was predicted to be bad for them, they had *huge* blood glucose swings and impaired glucose tolerance! When they followed the diet that was predicted to be good for them, however, they had *fully normalized* blood glucose levels for the entire week. Wow! The bad diet gave them a prediabetic glucose response profile, while the good diet gave them a perfectly normal and healthy blood glucose response.

This study illustrates that there really is no such thing as a universal diet that works for all people! Scientifically, we see that our bodies really do respond differently to different foods. And when your friend did really well on a certain diet but you tried it and you didn't lose a pound? Now you can see that it was likely the right diet for your friend's body but the exact wrong diet for *you*!

These are not the only scientists working on this concept, by the way. One of my favorite researchers (and writers), Dr. Tim Spector, is also doing research on personalized nutrition.[5] In 2019, his team released a groundbreaking study that compared individual responses to foods of 1,100 adults from the United States and the UK, and within this group, there was something else interesting: 60 percent of the subjects were *twins*. You see, Dr. Spector is interested in not only how the gut microbiome affects our personal responses to foods but also what role genetics might play. Who better to study than twins?

Spector and his team have been studying twins for years, and he is most famous for his work on a twenty-five-year investigation called the Twins UK Study. In his work, he explores how much of the similarities and differences between two people might be related to genetics, and how much might be related to other factors.

In their most recent study, which they called PREDICT, they measured blood glucose, insulin levels, fat levels (triglycerides), and other blood markers in response to a variety of meals.[6] Just as Dr. Segal's group found in the previous study, Spector's group found that there was a wide variation in responses to the same exact meals. Some of the participants had blood sugar and insulin spikes, while others had fat levels that hung around in their bloodstreams for hours after they had eaten.

Genetic factors explained some of the variation in responses, but not most of it; just under 50 percent of the blood glucose differences were linked to genetics, while 30 percent of the differences in insulin response and 20 percent of the difference in triglycerides were related to genetics. Much of the difference was again attributed to variations in gut microbiome composition, just as Dr. Segal's work found. Identical twins, though identical genetically, have only a 37 percent similarity in their gut microbiome compositions.

Now, the team is working on a second study called PREDICT 2, which will include thousands of new participants as they refine their predictive algorithms even more.

Y'all, we are at a turning point in nutritional understanding here! This PREDICT information is hot off the presses (at the time that I am writing this, it has been out for less than two months). While this science is still in its infancy, I predict that we will see more and more about bio-individuality over the coming years as companies explore both the genetic and gut-microbiome relationships to our individual "ideal" diets.[7]

How can we use this information *now*? Depending upon when you read this book, perhaps more research will have been done and it'll be common knowledge that we all have differences in what foods work best for us individually. Right now in 2020, however, that isn't true, so you may have to be a bit of a detective to figure it out. When you want to determine what foods work well for your body, one strategy is to think back over your own diet history. Which diet worked the best for *your* body in the past? That may give you a clue.

Here's how this looks for me. As I have mentioned in earlier chapters, I tried *all* the diets over the years. When I look back at my results, I have now realized that I never did lose weight following a low-carb approach, even though I tried to be low-carb over and over, in all the different variations that hit the market (Atkins, Suzanne Somers, Carbohydrate Addicts, keto). Even when I stuck to one of those plans for *months,* I never lost any weight. (Why did I keep trying and trying something that clearly didn't work for my body? The theories were so compelling! I *knew* it would work if I just tried hard enough. Except it never did work for me.)

What *did* work for me was the low-fat diet of the 1990s. As long as I stuck to it, I was able to remain slim without counting a single calorie . . . all I counted were fat grams. While I soon got tired of living that way (fat-free products are disgusting, and I love butter), there is no question that this style of eating worked for my body.

I'm currently at what feels like my ideal weight, so I don't *need* to lose any more weight. While I still have some cellulite hanging around and I will never be a bikini model, I am able to eat the foods I love every day (even my beloved butter) without restriction, and I'm okay with having a little extra fluff here and there, if it means I get to eat foods that are delicious. I'm currently wearing a size 0–2, and that's good enough for me. If, however, I did want to shed some of that extra fluff, I would consider cutting back on some of the fat in my daily diet. Why? Because I remember my success from the 1990s, and I had my DNA analyzed to see if it provided any clues as to what foods might work best for my body.

First, I did a standard DNA analysis offered by one of the main players in the DNA testing world. Not only did I learn some fascinating things about my ancestry that I didn't know, I learned that I am likely to be an extremely restless sleeper (true!), I'm more likely to detect bitter flavors in foods (true!), and I am likely to use more caffeine than other people (Lordy, that's true!).

After examining the general information provided by the company, I took it one step further; I *downloaded* my raw data from their web platform and *uploaded* it to another company's web platform. The second company (and there are many others out there like the one I used) analyzes every bit of your raw data and generates a report with recommendations based on your complete profile.

As I've already said, please understand that this research is still in its infancy and that not all our bio-individuality is related to our genes; a good bit of it is related to our gut microbiomes and a genetic test can't tell you anything about your gut inhabitants. Still, my results are interesting and fit in with what I remember from my past dieting experience; my DNA analysis indicates that a lower-fat approach is recommended for my body, with a higher percentage of carbs and a moderate protein intake.

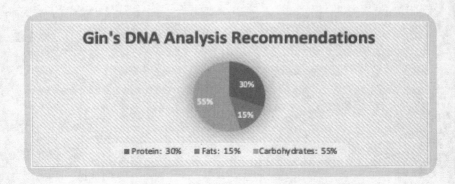

Gin's DNA Analysis Recommendations

30%

55%

15%

■ Protein: 30% ■ Fats: 15% ■ Carbohydrates: 55%

Looking at this graph, you can see why a high-fat keto plan may have not been the best fit for my body, but the low-fat diets of the 1990s worked well for me. High carbs for the win! In another brand-new study from 2019, scientists have found that approximately 50 percent of us have a gene that helps our bodies regulate blood glucose, meaning that we are physically adapted to a higher carb intake, but the other 50 percent of us don't have it.[8] The theory is that some of our ancestors developed this gene variant in response to the agricultural revolution, while others of us have the older gene variant. Since this study is so new, I don't know which variant I have, but I have a suspicion that I've got the newer one based on what I have discovered about the way my body reacts to carbs. If you have a hunch that *your* body does *not* react well to carbs, you're probably right about that one, too.

I look forward to the day when we have more research on this fascinating topic! You know I will be following it closely.

In the meantime, I hope that you have fully abandoned any traces of diet brain that you have been carrying around. Now you can see that it is foolish to search for the one perfect diet for everyone when we can see that there is absolutely no such thing after all!

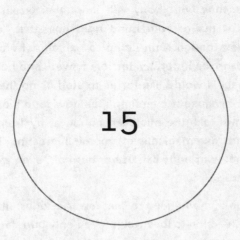

15

THE END OF THE CALORIE

Now that we have learned that there is no one best diet for all people, let's dig into another staple of the diet world: the common calorie! Everyone knows that if you eat less and move more, you'll lose weight, right? And we have all been taught that the best way to eat less is to count calories so that you know when to stop eating. Even better, you can find a very scientific formula that allows you to input personal data about yourself, and it will calculate exactly how many calories your body "needs" on a day-to-day basis. We have heard the good news that all we have to do is eat 500 calories per day below our bodies' maintenance requirements and we'll lose a pound per week. Yay for math!

Except that that's not how it works at all. Oops.

Let's unpack a few simple concepts first, because I want you to know a few things right off the bat:

- Yes, it's true that if you "eat more calories" than your body can use (or burn off, by increasing your metabolic rate), you'll gain weight, because your body will store the excess energy. (So, please get it out of your mind right now that "calories don't count." Even though I am going to explain why counting calories is an exercise in futility, terribly flawed, and I don't want you to do it—heck, I would like for us to stop using the word *calorie* altogether, because it oversimplifies how food works within the body—do not take the mistaken notion away from this chapter that the body can magically overcome overeating. If you overeat beyond what your body can use or burn off, even with IF, you will gain weight.)

- Yes, it's true that you need to "eat fewer calories" than your body requires to function to lose weight. You only burn fat for fuel if you have a *need* to access that energy! If you take in too much food, you won't *need* to access your stored fat.

BUT!

- NO, it's *not* true that our bodies process or use all calories the same way! You often hear that "a calorie is a calorie," but that is the biggest lie of all. That's one of the main reasons why the calories in / calories out model doesn't work. (One of the other main reasons has to do with the flaws in the "calories out" side of the equation, which I taught you in the introduction; recall the science of metabolic adaptation, which is why "calories out" never does work out in our favor when we over-restrict long term.)

- NO, it's *not* true that counting calories is the best method to figure out how much energy your body can extract from the foods you eat! As I have already taught you, the body is amazingly adaptable and can turn *down* your metabolic rate in response to over-restriction and can turn *up* your metabolic rate in response to overfeeding. It's impossible to take these complex metabolic adaptations into account with any formula, and it's the reason why people fail to lose weight as mathematically predicted when they are following a calorie-counting protocol.

Hopefully, I will convince you that you'll never need (or even want) to count another calorie. Yep. It's true. Your body isn't going to process 100 calories of almonds in the same way it processes 100 calories of sugary soda, so why would you even bother tallying up your calories? In addition, I will discuss the pitfalls of calorie counting and how we can once and for all free ourselves from the calorie-counting madness. (Spoiler alert: counting calories to control your intake actually makes it *harder* to reconnect with your body's satiety signals!)

Where did the concept of counting calories in foods come from, anyway? Let's have a history lesson!

From what we can tell, the first use of the word *calorie* came in 1825 in a French scientific journal.[1] A couple of chemists were studying energy with a goal of calculating the amount of work that could be performed by a steam engine, and they used the idea of a calorie to represent the amount of heat energy required to raise the temperature of water by one degree. Then, in the 1890s, a chemist named Wilbur Atwater wanted to figure out how to apply this information to foods with the goal of helping the poor make the most of their food choices. Isn't it interesting how the pendulum has swung in the other direction? His work was begun to combat malnutrition, and now we most frequently think of calories in the concept of *over*nutrition.

To calculate how many calories are in a common food, you start with a tool called a *bomb calorimeter*. First, insert the food into a container that is surrounded by water and heat it until the food is fully burned off. By measuring the change in the temperature of the water, the number of calories in that food can be determined. Atwater knew, however, that our bodies "lose" some of the energy from a food through our various waste products (urine, poop, heat . . .). He came up with a simple formula:

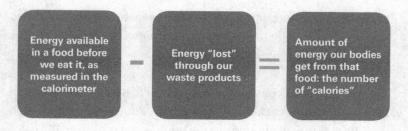

Technically, when we refer to a *calorie* (such as on a food label), we are really talking about kilocalories, but in general use, we use the term *calorie* to discuss the energy from food, so you don't need to worry about the specifics of kilocalorie versus calorie.

Through these methods, Atwater discovered that carbohydrates and protein have about four calories per gram, fat has about nine calories per gram, and alcohol has about seven calories per gram.

While Atwater realized that our bodies are more complicated than a bomb calorimeter, his formula is still a huge oversimplification of what goes on within the body—but we are still using his calculations today! Modern-day calorie values for foods are calculated by taking the number of grams of each macronutrient found in the food (protein, carbohydrate, fat, alcohol) and multiplying the amounts by the number of calories in a standard gram of that nutrient (four, nine, or seven).

You may be surprised to learn that our bodies process foods very differently from the way Atwater predicted, however, so we extract wildly different amounts of energy from the foods than the calorie label actually indicates. Newer science reveals that standard calorie counts have some serious flaws, and it has to do with the way our bodies digest our foods and extract the usable energy:

- Our bodies get *more* energy from foods that have been cooked versus foods that are raw! As an example, your body has to do more work to digest raw spinach than cooked spinach, so you'll "waste" more of the energy found in the raw spinach as your body breaks down the leaves and the stems. This is also true for meats, and we get more energy from cooked meats than raw meats (though this doesn't mean I am asking you to go on a raw-meat diet).[2]

You see, cooking changes the structure of our foods and makes the energy more easily accessible, so rather than our bodies having to do all the digestive work, that work is done by the heat of the cooking process. A steak tartare, therefore, would have fewer accessible calories than a well-done steak, even if they started out with the same number of theoretical calories.

- Our bodies use more energy processing whole foods than processed foods! So, eating 100 calories of carrots will cause us to "waste" more of that energy on the digestion process than when we eat 100 calories of carrot cake. In one study, scientists compared two different cheese sandwiches: one that was made from highly processed bread and cheese and another that was made from more "whole" versions. It took almost 47 percent *more* energy to digest the less processed version of the sandwich, and the metabolic rates of the participants went *up* as they digested the meal![3]

  Processed foods have easily accessible energy that are already broken down for us through the processing itself. Thinking about that same well-done steak from the previous example; that steak would have fewer accessible calories than a well-done hamburger patty, since the hamburger has been ground into small pieces—less work for your body to do equals more "calories" available to you, even though the two food items may have the same amount of "energy" within the meat itself.

- Nuts are particularly problematic when it comes to the accuracy of stated calorie counts. Raw peanuts provide fewer "calories" to the body than roasted peanut butter.[4] When we eat almonds, rather than 170 calories per serving, as listed on the label, our bodies can only extract 129 calories of usable energy.[5] A similar result has been found for both pistachios and walnuts.[6] Because the cell walls of these foods reduce digestibility, even the fats found in these nuts

tend to make it out the other side of the body without being accessed. (The study authors describe the consumption of nuts as
leading to "increased fecal weight and fat content" after eating
nuts, and even while typing that, I am glad I am not a scientist per-
forming nut-digestion studies.)

So, we see that all foods aren't processed the same way within our
bodies, and this can make a huge difference in how many calories
are available to us. But did you know that even if two people eat the
exact same foods, not everyone is going to get the same number of
calories from their foods? Both the length of your intestinal tract and
the composition of your gut microbiomes affect how many calories
your body extracts from those foods, and those are just two of the
personal factors that affect digestion (more proof that we really are
all different when it comes to what foods work well for our bodies!).

If all of this weren't enough to convince you to kick calorie counting to the curb, did you know that some foods are more likely to be
stored as fat than others? In one study, when subjects were overfed
either fats or carbohydrates for fourteen days, scientists found that
participants only stored 75–85 percent of the excess energy when
they were overfed carbohydrates, but they stored 90–95 percent of
the excess energy when they were overfed fats.[7] Another study
explains why that happened. In the second study, participants who
were overfed carbohydrates had an increase in their twenty-four-
hour energy expenditure of 7 percent, while those who were overfed
fat didn't have any increase in energy expenditure.[8]

This science all goes together to teach us one thing: the most important factor is what your body *does with the foods you eat,* not how many
calories are on the label. Some foods require more effort for your body
to process, and you'll "lose" calories to the digestive process. Some
foods cause your body to ramp up energy expenditure because they
aren't easy to store, while others are more easily processed and stored
on your body as fat. And some *bodies* process foods more efficiently
than other bodies.

What's a calorie counter to do?

I remember my own ventures into calorie counting from decades past. I read somewhere that I should eat 1,200 calories each day to lose weight. Every day, I would portion out those 1,200 calories so I could have small amounts of food at regular intervals. It was so difficult to get through the day; I was constantly starving! Because I kept my body in the fed state with the frequent, small amounts of food, I wasn't tapping into my fat stores effectively, which explains why I was so miserable (and why low-calorie diets that have you eating frequently throughout the day fail . . . most of us can't take it for long). This is very different from the way I feel when I live an intermittent fasting lifestyle. It's so easy to fast when I am well fueled by my body fat! Then I get to enjoy a satisfying amount of food every evening!

So, we all know that all-day, low-calorie dieting is a recipe for failure. Let's say, however, that I decided I would pair low-calorie dieting with intermittent fasting and count calories within my eating window, just to make sure that I'm not over- or under-eating. What could be wrong with that approach? A lot, actually.

Even though we have just learned that calorie counts are meaningless because what really matters is what our bodies do with the foods we eat, some long-term dieters may still be reluctant to let the practice of counting calories go. You may worry that without tracking what you eat, you'll go nuts and eat everything in sight, with no Off switch. (Of course, as I mentioned in the FAST Start chapter, don't fret if this happens at first. It's typical to overeat as your body adapts to IF.) Or you may worry that you won't eat *enough* and will inadvertently slow your metabolic rate. It can be difficult to give up calorie counting if you think it is helping you!

Even if we ignore the flaws with calorie counting that I have taught you in this chapter, there are two other reasons why I don't want you to count calories:

1. Metabolic adaptation! I have taught you about this concept in earlier chapters. Whenever we do something that is exactly the

same day in and day out, our bodies are more likely to adapt. So, if you decide that you want to count your calories and eat to a predetermined calorie target day after day, you are at more risk of metabolic adaptation than someone who naturally varies the amount of foods eaten from day to day.

2. Counting calories teaches us to rely on *external cues* to decide how much we eat rather than trusting our *internal cues*.

In the next chapter on appetite correction, I am going to explain how our hunger and satiety signals work and why we can trust these signals from our bodies as we determine how much food we require in a given day.

The *only time* I give you reluctant permission to count calories is if you are following the up-and-down-day IF protocol, and in that case, I *only* want you to count calories on the down days (unless you are doing the full-fast version, in which case it is easy to count to zero). Even though calorie counting is flawed, the point of the down days is to purposefully cycle through the down pattern while eating without restriction on the up days. If you can't remember why this is helpful, go back and reread chapter 7. I know it may be confusing for me to tell you that counting calories is flawed and then tell you that I still want you to do it as a part of your down-day IF protocol, and I'm sorry for that. I wish there were another way to manage down-day intake other than calorie counting, but there just isn't. Hopefully, you'll realize that it's a necessary evil and you'll forgive me, especially when you're having stunning success with IF.

So! Let's learn about appetite correction, which is the magical tool that will free you from counting calories forever!

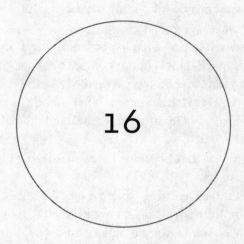

16

APPETITE CORRECTION: WHAT EXACTLY IS THIS HORMONAL VOODOO?

When I was obese, I was always in search of a better way to lose weight. I was weary after all the years of calorie and macro counting (what I was counting depended on whether I was low fat or low carb at the time), and I absolutely didn't want to count or track anything, ever again. One lucky day, I discovered the concept of intuitive eating.

I was entranced by the philosophy. The intuitive-eating approach promises that we can learn how to eat based on our natural hunger and satiety cues by giving ourselves unconditional permission to eat whenever we are hungry.[1] Over time, our bodies should self-regulate, allowing us to achieve our ideal weight without struggle.

It sounded absolutely perfect to me, weary as I was. I fully committed! I read the books. I drank the Kool-Aid (only when thirsty, of course!). As recommended, I put my scale away, and I waited for the magic to happen.

Unfortunately, that isn't what happened for me. I understood that I *should* be able to tell if I was hungry or not, but I just couldn't! Every time I asked myself, *Am I hungry?*, it seemed like the answer was, *Yes!* Still, I followed the guidelines, month after month, as my clothes got tighter. In my heart *and* in my head, I *so* wanted this to be the answer for me!

And the result is that I became more obese than I had ever been before!

Why didn't intuitive eating work for me? Now that I understand more about how the body works, I have a hunch that over time, I had lost the ability to *hear* leptin, my satiety hormone. Just as too much insulin leads us to develop insulin resistance, too much leptin leads to leptin resistance.[2] It's not that I didn't have *enough* leptin; it's that my body was no longer listening to it.

Here's what is exciting, though. Now that I am an intermittent faster, I absolutely understand what the intuitive-eating proponents had been talking about all along. *Finally,* I can understand the difference between *actual* hunger and the feeling of "I would *like* to eat now." I am certain that intermittent fasting has allowed my body to reconnect with both my hunger and my satiety signals in a way that had been lost to me when I was obese and eating frequently throughout the day.

Enter the concept of appetite correction!

Appetite correction is a term coined by Dr. Bert Herring, who developed the Fast-5 intermittent fasting plan that was my introduction to the daily-eating-window approach all those years ago.

What does *appetite correction* mean? It means that you are back in tune with your body's appetite control center: the appestat. When you experience appetite correction, you don't need to count calories to know when you have had enough to eat; your body sends you the "stop eating" signals, *and* you can hear them. (Of course, you still have to *listen* to these signals. It's possible to override them and keep eating. If that happens, you'll likely wish you had stopped when you first got the signal. We have all been there, and after you feel that "Oops! I ate too much!" feeling a few times, you learn to listen more closely.)

What exactly is the appestat? Within the hypothalamus region of our brains, we have both a "satiety center" and a "feeding center," which make up our appestat. In early experiments, scientists were able to *increase* appetite (and weight) by damaging the area now known as the satiety center and *decrease* appetite (and weight) by damaging the feeding center.[3] This illustrated the connection between these two sections of the hypothalamus and appetite.

How does the appestat work? In theory, it works like your home's thermostat. When your body senses that you need to eat more food, it cranks up your hunger hormones and turns down your satiety hormones. The result is that you are hormonally driven to eat more food and don't feel easily satisfied. In contrast, when your body decides you have had enough, it can decrease your hunger hormones and increase satiety hormones so that you stop eating.

If you've ever spent time with a newborn baby, you have seen this in action. When a baby is hungry, no one can rest until that baby is fed! How does the baby *know* it is hungry? After all, the baby isn't counting calories. It's the appestat!

On the flip side, once a baby has had enough to eat, there is no way you are going to convince him to take in another drop. I remember trying to feed my older son, and he had this thing he did with his lips that was a clear signal that he was *not* going to have any more, no matter how much I tried to get him to. How did he *know* he had enough? Again, it's the appestat!

It's probably been a long time since you were able to hear your hunger and satiety signals as well as a newborn baby's. Keep one thing in mind—some people *never lose* their connections with their appestats! These are your friends and family members who have remained lean for their whole lives—the ones who you watch with amazement at holiday gatherings as they put down their forks with cake *still left on the plate.* We call those ~~annoying~~ lucky people "naturally thin," and my husband is one of them. He *always* knew how to stop eating when he'd had enough food, and he couldn't understand why I was unable to just do the same.

Somehow, along the way, however, the rest of us lose touch with the signals from our hunger and satiety hormones. There are many factors that cause this to happen, and here are just a few of them:

- We are taught to eat at mealtimes whether we are hungry or not, and our well-meaning mothers don't let us leave the table until we clean our plates.

- We follow weight-loss diets and learn to focus on external cues, such as calories, fat grams, and so on to tell us when we have had enough.

- Ultra-processed foods are highly palatable, and these foods disrupt our appetite control systems.[4] (I'll tell you more about this problem in the next chapter! Stay tuned.)

Once we lose touch with these signals, we have to work really hard to reconnect with them. The good news is that we absolutely can! I have, and I believe that you can, too.

I find Dr. Herring's concept of appetite correction to be the cornerstone to becoming a more intuitive eater *within the intermittent fasting framework.* Our goal is to learn to trust our bodies again (though first we may have to give our bodies time to trust *us* again, particularly if we have a long and complicated dieting history). This two-way trust can be regained, and I believe that intermittent fasting is the answer.

In the introduction, I taught you that when we follow an overly restrictive diet long term, our bodies adapt as a protective measure. Metabolic rate slows, and our bodies also send us "eat now!" signals.[5] This slowing of our metabolic rate leads to an increase in ghrelin (our hunger hormone) and a decrease in leptin (our satiety hormone), both designed to get us to eat the food our bodies think we need.

Does intermittent fasting help us reconnect with these signals? Dr. Herring believes so, as do thousands of intermittent fasters that I have worked with in my online intermittent fasting support communities. It's fun to watch brand-new intermittent fasters report that *they* are now the person leaving uneaten cake on their plates! Suddenly, we become able to hear the "stop eating now" signals loud and clear, and it's an incredible feeling.

We also have some brand-new research on this topic, which is exciting! In a 2019 study, scientists found that even after only *four days* of following a six-hour eating window, participants saw a reduction in ghrelin and an increase in leptin.[6] This was a very small study, the participants crammed all three of their typical meals into an early six-hour eating window, and four days is *nothing* (since we know it takes a lot longer for our bodies to adapt to IF), but it's still an affirmation of the stunning appetite correction that so many intermittent fasters report.

Keep one thing in mind: the process of appetite control is very complex, and control isn't limited to the hypothalamus (or to the actions of leptin and ghrelin, for that matter).[7] There are other hunger and satiety hormones besides leptin and ghrelin (neuropeptide Y, orexins, agouti-related peptide, cholecystokinin, glucagon-like peptide 1, and so on), but I focused on leptin and ghrelin in this chapter, since they are the ones that you'll hear about the most. For our purposes, all that matters is that we understand that our bodies send us signals through many pathways to help regulate how much we eat and that intermittent fasting helps us reconnect with these signals.

Here's something to also understand about appetite correction: it works both ways! Sometimes, IFers think appetite correction only means that we get full quickly and find it easy to stop when satisfied. That's part of it, but it's not the end of the story! Some days, you'll have an *increased* appetite. Listen to your body! Increased hunger on some days is also a feature of appetite correction. Once we understand this fact, we can be a lot easier on ourselves when we have a hungrier day. It's not just because you are *weak* or *bad* or a glutton. No, hormones are powerful things, and it's hard to resist their mighty signals!

When we learn to listen to our bodies, we don't need to count calories or track macros. We trust our satiety (and hunger) signals, and we *stop when satisfied* (or eat more when we need to).

It's so important to never forget this one fact, though—when you are trying to lose weight, the amount you eat *does* matter. Your goal is to *stop when satisfied* and not to keep eating more just because your window is still open. You want to *stop when satisfied,* not overly full. You know that Thanksgiving Day overstuffed feeling? That's how you feel when you eat too much. We don't want to get to that point. *Stop when satisfied.*

I keep repeating those words: **Stop when satisfied.**

This can be a difficult thing for new intermittent fasters who are trying to embrace the concept of appetite correction but aren't there yet. Maybe you are not in tune with your satiety signals yet, and it's going to take awhile longer for you. Maybe you *hear* them, but you still aren't good at *listening* to them. Until you reach the state where your satiety cues are normalized, you may need coping strategies to prevent overeating.

In Okinawa, Japan, residents are known for living long and healthy lives, and they follow a philosophy known as *hara hachi bu.* This phrase is based on a teaching by Confucius, and it means "eat until 80 percent full." Keep this phrase in the back of your mind while you are eating. You don't want to be completely full, simply pleasantly satisfied. To put it another way, stop eating when you are *no longer hungry.*

There's one sign that many of us have when we've had enough to eat: the sigh. Have you ever been eating a meal, and then experienced a sigh of satisfaction? I want you to start paying attention to that feeling. It is one way our bodies tell us that we have had enough.

When you feel the sigh, stop eating. Give your body time to check in with your feelings of satiety. In a few minutes, you may recognize that you have, indeed, had enough to eat. It's a powerful feeling to realize that your body communicated to you and you listened!

Whenever I ignore that "I've had enough" sigh and keep eating (face it: food is delicious!), I am usually sorry about fifteen minutes later. It reinforces the fact that it's best to pay attention! You can always go back and eat more later if you truly haven't had enough, but once you have overdone it, you're stuck with that overstuffed feeling.

Another sign that you have had enough to eat is that food starts to taste slightly less delicious. I know that may sound weird, but start paying attention to this as you eat. When your food starts to taste less delicious, stop eating and give your body a few minutes to check in with your satiety signals. You may find that you have had enough, and you'll be glad you were paying attention.

If you still need a little help with this concept as your body learns to listen to your satiety signals, I have a trick you can use.

When it's time to eat, serve yourself a plate of food *slightly smaller* than you think you need. If you finish that plate of food and you're still hungry, walk away from the table and set a timer for thirty minutes. Tell yourself that if you are still hungry when the timer goes off, you can have seconds. Usually what happens is that your body has time to register that you've had enough, and when the timer goes off, you will realize that you don't need any more food.

Eventually, you'll become better at recognizing when you've had enough. You won't need coping strategies, and you'll realize with delight that you have become an intuitively eating intermittent faster, just as I am now.

Also, never forget this important lesson: increased hunger that continues over time is a sign of metabolic adaptation that we should pay attention to.[8] Remember—everything that happens in our bodies is designed to protect us and keep us alive so we can reproduce. Don't ignore hunger that is getting worse and worse over time. If your body is sending you "eat more food" messages, make a change in your intermittent fasting protocol. Maybe it's time for you to do ADF for a while . . . the up days might be just what your body needs!

I've talked a lot about satiety in this chapter, and satiety is also related to food quality. When we select real foods that are full of nutrients, our bodies are happy and satisfied. More about this in the next chapter!

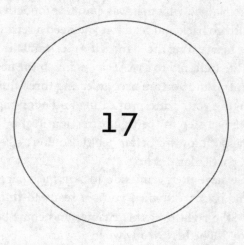

17

BEANS VS. JELLY BEANS: DOES FOOD QUALITY MATTER?

Spoiler alert: YES! Food quality does matter! We all understand that beans are actual food and jelly beans are candy. One will provide nutrients to your body, and the other is what we call *empty calories*.

This chapter will get into the science of processed foods versus whole foods and why what we eat matters to our bodies. Be careful, though—we don't want to turn our diet brains back on; that isn't the goal at all! By making a few simple tweaks, we can nudge ourselves closer to the "real food" side of the continuum without becoming obsessed or overly dogmatic about what we eat.

Before we get into this topic, however, I want to get one thing out into the open. Remember the FAST Start, where I told you that you shouldn't try to change *what* you are eating during your first twenty-eight days? I meant that. Please don't think you need to jump right into intermittent fasting *and* do a total overhaul of what you're eating all at once. I explained why that was counterproductive in the FAST Start section, so go back and read it if you need a refresher.

If you have been eating the Standard American Diet for a while, or most of your life (referred to as *SAD* by many in the health and wellness community), and you are used to eating three times a day (plus snacks), changing your pattern of eating and adopting intermittent fasting is already a step in the right direction! Just by beginning IF, you are on the path toward better health, so don't stress about what you're eating, particularly at first.

In fact, you have my permission to *skip this chapter entirely* for now and come back to it when you are ready to think about food choices. Yep. Skip right over this chapter and come back to it later. Not a problem! I'll be here, ready when you are.

You'll have plenty of time to figure out what foods work for your body over the coming months and years, and it's almost universal that those of us who live an intermittent fasting lifestyle find that our tastes completely change over time. So, today you may crave fast food and packaged snack foods, but in a year, I predict you will be *shocked* at how little those things appeal to you. The first time you find that your previously favorite "treat" tastes gross to you, you will probably do what I did—accuse the company of changing their recipe. Nope! They didn't change; *you* did.

Just as I have taught you to listen to your body when it comes to *how much* to eat, I want to teach you to listen to your body when it comes to *what* to eat. When you remember that we are all different when it comes to what foods work best for our bodies, you can turn off your diet brain and tune in to your inner wisdom.

Here's an example of how that worked for me. Over time, I have realized that I don't feel great when I eat sugar. For years, I have suffered from restless legs, and this began well before intermittent fasting. Thanks to IF, however, I have become connected to my body in a new way, and so I have been able to figure out that for me, eating too much sugar leads to restless legs and the inability to get a good night's sleep.

Do I avoid sugar 100 percent of the time? No. Am I a lot choosier about how much sugar I'll eat? Absolutely. Just the other day, I was craving a peanut butter milkshake from my favorite ice cream shop in town. I thought about driving over there to get one. Then I thought about how I would feel after drinking it. Was it worth having restless legs for the rest of the evening? I decided it was not, so I didn't go get it. Boom! I was completely in charge at all times. I could have made the other choice, and there are days where I do choose to eat something sugary. I don't feel guilty or beat myself up when I do, but I do accept that I may not feel my best.

This is a powerful concept to wrap your brain around. I don't avoid sugar because I read a book or watched a video that told me sugar was "bad." Instead, I learned to listen to my body and connect the way I feel to what I eat. This is the power of intermittent fasting. I *can* have whatever I want, but now I am better equipped to figure out what I *actually* want. And what I want most of all is to feel great. So, I make (most of!) my decisions accordingly. If I am going to have cake or ice cream, however, I make sure it is really high quality and delicious and worth every bite. I'm certainly not going to choose grocery store cake or cheap ice cream. Those are easy to pass up, as they are not window-worthy.

Now that I've gotten that out of the way, let's learn about food!

You've probably heard people say that we should avoid processed foods and stick to real foods. Heck, I've even used that terminology here within this book, especially when I mentioned the time in 2015 where I temporarily delayed processed foods to reach my goals more quickly. The word *processed*, however, can be confusing. Let me explain.

I have gotten into making my own bread from scratch, and I feel like some kind of magician every time I do it. I start with organic whole-wheat grains, grind them into flour using a grain mill, mix up bread dough, and bake delicious homemade bread. The bread I make from the flour I mill at home retains all the fiber, nutrients, and enzymes from the wheat grains, yet it is still processed because I ground it into flour using the grain mill. Of course, this is *very* different from the white flour I could buy in the store, where all the good stuff has been removed. The flour in the store is a lot more processed than the flour I make at home, but both have technically been processed. Clearly, we need another term besides *processed* to understand when too much processing becomes a problem. Luckily, we have it.

The new term that you'll hear being used is *ultra-processed*.

Ultra-processed foods are one of the biggest problems of the modern era. Higher consumption of these products is associated with many (if not most) of the modern lifestyle diseases, and this is a worldwide problem.[1]

In 2016, the UN designated the years 2016–2025 as the Decade of Nutrition.[2] In support of these initiatives, the Global Panel on Agriculture and Food Systems for Nutrition released a report identifying the modern challenges faced by the world. In it, you'll find this definition:

> The term "ultra-processed" was coined to refer to industrial formulations manufactured from substances derived from foods or synthesized from other organic sources. They typically contain little or no whole foods, are ready-to-consume or heat up, and are fatty, salty, or sugary and depleted in dietary fibre, protein, various micronutrients and other bioactive compounds. Examples include: sweet, fatty, or salty packaged snack products, ice cream, sugar-sweetened beverages, chocolates, confectionery, French fries, burgers and hot dogs, and poultry and fish nuggets.[3]

Many of these products give us the impression that they are healthy by the way they are packaged or labeled. You can go down the breakfast cereal aisle, as an example, and find the sugary cereals marketed as "contains whole grains!" or "all of the vitamins and minerals you need!"

Can I tell you a really embarrassing story? When my boys were little, I fed them a chocolate-flavored food-like beverage in their sippy cups every single day. I was young, and I didn't know anything about nutrition, but I did know that this product was chock-full of vitamins and minerals, so I thought I was doing something *good* for my kids. Sigh. I was taken in by the claims, too. I thought it was a better choice than *actual milk*.

The good news is that there is a new classification system that will help us make sense of how far along the continuum—from "unprocessed" to "ultra-processed"—various foods fall. It's called the NOVA food classification, and I predict we will be hearing more about it in coming years.[4]

Here are the four groups from the NOVA food classification system:

CATEGORY	GROUP 1 UNPROCESSED OR MINIMALLY PROCESSED FOODS	GROUP 2 PROCESSED CULINARY INGREDIENTS	GROUP 3 PROCESSED FOODS	GROUP 4 ULTRA-PROCESSED FOODS
Simple Description	Fresh foods that come from plants or animals with little processing.	Other culinary ingredients that we use in our cooking.	Foods made from a combination of fresh foods and culinary items.	Products made with little to no fresh food content with a large quantity of refined and processed additives.
More Information	These foods are the edible parts of plants (the seeds, fruits, leaves, stems, or roots) and animals (meat, dairy, eggs). Foods fit into this category if they have had inedible or unwanted parts removed or if they have been crushed	These ingredients come from the foods in group 1, and they are derived from substances from nature. Foods from this category may have been pressed, refined, ground, milled, or dried. These ingredients are	These foods have been made by combining items from group 1 and group 2. Processes include a wide variety of preservation and/or cooking methods, including fermentation. Most of these foods contain two or three	These products are formulations made either mostly or entirely from substances derived from foods and not the foods themselves. They also include chemical additives. Overall, you find very little actual "food" from group 1 within these products. Many of the ingredients may sound like food,

cont.

	or dried for the purpose of preservation, storage, or to make them safe or edible.	not stand-alone food but are used in combination with foods from group 1 by home cooks.	ingredients and still remain recognizable as versions of foods from group 1.	such as casein, lactose, whey, gluten, and hydrogenated oils. You'll also find preservatives, stabilizers, dyes, artificial flavors, etc.
Examples	Fresh fruits and vegetables, whole grains, milk, eggs, meat	Oils, butter, flour, sugar, honey, salt	Homemade bread, cheese, canned goods	Most bottled and canned beverages, sweet or savory packaged snacks, meat products (like hot dogs), frozen meals, canned meals

As you can see, the bread that I make at home would fall into category 3: processed. I start with some items from category 1 (whole wheat, milk, yeast, and an egg), add in some items from category 2 (salt and honey), and end up with my homemade bread. In contrast, the bread I would buy at the grocery store in the bread aisle would fit into category 4: ultra-processed, with a long list of ingredients.

You can use the NOVA classification to help you make choices about what foods to emphasize. It's simple—select mostly items from the first three categories, and limit items from the ultra-processed column.

You can also think of it this way: If we went back in time to before the Industrial Revolution and sat down with our great-great-great grandparents, what foods would have been available to them? Most of the foods that you eat on a day-to-day basis should be actual foods that they would recognize. Eat *mostly* those foods.

One of the problems with the foods from the ultra-processed column is that they have been designed to be hyperpalatable, meaning you "can't eat just one." (Remember that line from the popular commercial? They aren't kidding!) These foods are also convenient, last a long time on the shelf, and are not only cheap for you to purchase but highly profitable for the food manufacturers.

When you eat a diet that is high in ultra-processed foods, you end up overfed and yet undernourished. In this instance, obesity is a form of malnutrition![5] I know that sounds counterintuitive; if someone is overweight, they have taken in *too much food*. That is true. But you can eat large quantities of ultra-processed foods and receive very few nutrients. Even though you may be carrying around dozens of extra pounds of fat, your body is literally starving for nutrition.

How does this happen? These ultra-processed foods drive you to *eat more food*.[6] You see, our bodies don't count calories; they count *nutrients*.

When you eat a diet that is made up of mostly ultra-processed foods, this is what happens. You eat. Your body realizes that you haven't provided necessary nutrients and sends you a message: "That wasn't it. Send something else down." So, you eat again. "Nope. That still wasn't it. Try again." You eat something else. "Still no! Keep trying!"

Have you ever felt trapped in that type of vicious cycle? You're eating and eating and yet not satisfied?

Now you are equipped to understand why that happens. If you eat and eat and aren't satisfied, think about *what* you have eaten. Have you provided your body with sufficient nutrients? If not, now you know what to do! Send down some high-quality foods and see what your body thinks then.

For me, the difference is striking. I used to eat at McDonald's frequently, and we had dinner from the drive-through at least once a week. Because I truly don't demonize any foods (even now), I decided on a particularly rushed day that I would enjoy my favorite McDonald's meal, guilt-free: a Big Mac and large fries, with a Coke. If you're a calorie counter, you would know that this meal contains about 1,340 calories, according to the nutrition information provided from McDonald's. After I ate the meal, I was full.

A couple of hours later, I found myself in the kitchen, aimlessly wandering around, looking for something to eat. Have you ever done that? I kept eating different things and remained completely unsatisfied. It was probably pretty funny to watch me randomly stuffing things into my mouth. Eventually, I felt overly full and yet *still* completely unsatisfied.

You see, it isn't about calories. It's about *nutrients.*

I had plenty of calories from that Big Mac meal and all the random things I'd eaten while wandering around the kitchen. And yet, I never got the signal from my body telling me I had eaten enough food.

Research shows that a diet high in ultra-processed foods causes us to eat approximately 500 more calories per day versus an unprocessed diet![7] One reason is that these foods disrupt our bodies' natural satiety signals and even can lead to addiction by activating the same reward pathways seen in drugs of abuse.[8] So, if you've ever felt like you're addicted to some of these foods, there is scientific evidence to support that you actually *are.*

In addition to driving us to eat more, there's another problem with ultra-processed foods. As I mentioned in the last chapter, our bodies can extract more calories from foods that are highly processed because we don't have to work as hard to digest those foods. So, 100 calories of jelly beans will be digested with little effort from our bodies, while 100 calories of actual beans will require a lot more energy to process.

What we want to do, then, is provide our bodies with sufficient nutrients so that our bodies know we are well nourished. That helps us get the "I've had enough!" message, which teaches us to stop eating after an appropriate amount of food. Upping our food quality helps us find the magical appetite correction that we are looking for, and you don't have to be "perfect" to experience these benefits. Start by adding in highly nutritious foods to every meal. Just by doing that, you'll increase satisfaction and be more likely to know when you have had enough to eat.

It's also easy to make a few simple tweaks at the grocery store that make a huge impact on your overall food quality. I know you have heard this before—shop mostly in the perimeter of the grocery store, and buy fewer things from the center aisles. Now you understand why this is so important! The meat counter, the produce section, and maybe even the bakery (if your grocery store makes homemade bread with a few simple ingredients) are your best options for high-quality foods. You'll need some things from the center aisles (olive oil, salt, flour, etc.) for cooking, and you may even want to toss in a few of your favorite ultra-processed foods. But the *majority* of your cart should not be full of ultra-processed items.

Also, become a label reader and compare products. When you are choosing between two ultra-processed foods, select the one that has fewer ingredients and only ones that you can (mostly) pronounce.

As an example, I'm not asking you to give up crackers entirely! I love crackers, particularly with cheese. Yes, crackers are an ultra-processed food. That doesn't mean you need to make your own homemade crackers or form a substitute made from cauliflower. When I choose crackers, these are my criteria:

- Must be delicious.

- Must contain fewer ingredients than the *more* ultra-processed varieties.

And that's it. I like to keep it simple!

And remember that we are *not* trying to turn our diet brains back on. If you find that you are becoming obsessed with reading the labels or making sure your food is "good enough" for you, take a step back. The goal is to feel great in your body, to choose foods that you love (and make you happy), and to live an enjoyable lifestyle. Some days, you'll still go through the drive-through . . . and that's okay!

PART III

REPEAT.

As the title of the book implies, intermittent fasting is simple: Fast. Feast. Repeat. Part 3 of *Fast. Feast. Repeat.* explores everything you will need to know to bring it all together so that intermittent fasting becomes your forever lifestyle. How do we shift our thinking from "diet" to "lifestyle"? What are the best methods to measure progress? How can our mind-sets make a difference? What's the role of exercise? How can we continue to tweak our intermittent fasting protocols and food choices over time if weight loss slows down? What does maintenance look like? I've got you covered with answers to all these questions, plus more!

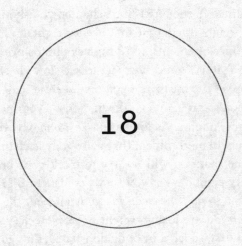

18

SCALE-SCHMALE: THE ULTIMATE GUIDE TO TRACKING YOUR PROGRESS

While I have already told you that intermittent fasting is the health plan with a side effect of weight loss, I get it; most of us—me included—came to intermittent fasting initially as a way to lose weight. And most of us are looking for an accurate and reliable way to measure our progress. In this chapter, I am going to give you a whole toolbox full of strategies for tracking your results so that you will know whether you are making measurable progress (of one kind or another) or not. And if you are not, you will know it for sure, thanks to these tools; no need to guess, y'all. Knowledge is power!

Unless you are on team no-scale (which I will explain in a minute), you will track your weight daily starting on day 29, *after* your body has had twenty-eight days to adjust to IF. (Don't forget that the initial weight you recorded on day 0 was for informational purposes only, and as I explained in the FAST Start chapter, you shouldn't expect to have lost any weight during the first twenty-eight days.) You will also begin taking measurements and progress photos every other week. After the FAST Start, you can expect to see slow yet steady progress in one or more of the measures: you may see the scale go down, you may see your measurements go down, and/or you may see changes in your progress photos. As long as *at least one* of these measures is changing, you will be confident that your body is changing!

Promise me that you will *not* try to track your progress during the first twenty-eight days as your body adjusts to IF! I mean it, y'all. That is the time to *nail the clean fast only* and *not* the time to stress about whether you are losing weight or not. Heck, you might even gain weight at first, so let your body do whatever it's going to do during those first few weeks without your constant attention on it.

Let's talk about all the tracking tools you'll have in your toolbox, and we need to start with the scale. Love it or hate it, the scale is the most common tool for most people who are trying to lose weight, and unfortunately, it's also one of the absolute *worst* tools for intermittent fasters! Why? There's a little thing that happens with IF called *body recomposition* (which is actually a *big* thing, and it is thrilling when you understand it).

As we learned in earlier chapters, when you are fasting clean, your body preferentially taps into fat stores for fuel during the fast. At the same time, your body ramps up human growth hormone (HGH) levels, meaning that your body is primed to build muscle like never before. Even if you aren't doing any official working out, you're moving your body throughout the day, and so your body is able to build muscle. (This confuses many people who think you have to be doing formal exercise to build muscle, but remember what I've already told you—babies and toddlers don't lift weights at the gym, but they build muscle tissue. Boom. So do you, thanks to the increases in HGH.)

Because we are tapping into our fat-burning superpower and also building muscle, we won't have the typical quick weight loss on the scale that you have probably had on diets you did in the past. IF is very different! This phenomenon causes a lot of angst among IFers who rely only on the scale to measure progress. They'll find that they are losing clothing sizes, but scale weight isn't changing at all. If the scale is your only measurement tool, you may think you aren't making any progress, when the opposite is true.

It's important to understand how body recomposition works. As you lose fat and build muscle, you will be getting smaller in size. This is because lean muscle takes up less space than the fluffy fat that you lost. To understand this, imagine some whipped margarine next to a sleek cut of filet mignon. The filet mignon (lean tissue) is more dense than the margarine (fat). If you had an equal volume of each (think of an amount of each that's the size of a pack of playing cards), you can imagine that the steak would weigh more than the margarine.

By the way, if you want to annoy a lot of people, make the statement that "muscle weighs more than fat." The sticklers in the crowd will tell you that a pound of muscle weighs the exact same amount as a pound of fat, which is true, but it misses the point. The truth is that *by volume,* muscle absolutely does weigh more than fat. If you had two equal-sized cubes the size of a Rubik's Cube and one was made of lead and one was made of Styrofoam, they would be the same volume, but the lead cube would weigh more. So, it's a fact that *by volume,* lead weighs more than Styrofoam. The same thing is true for muscle and fat; by volume, muscle weighs more than fat. The difference between lead and Styrofoam is more pronounced than the difference between muscle and fat, but hopefully, this example illustrates the point.

So, if you are experiencing this phenomenon, always trust your changing size more than you trust the scale! If you are getting measurably smaller and the scale isn't changing, you now know it is body recomposition in action. And NO—the fat isn't "turning into" muscle. They are two separate processes, but they are happening during the same period.

After understanding how the scale can be a liar, you may be tempted to throw your scale away entirely, and that's perfectly acceptable. I do think it's important to have *some* sort of measurement tools in your tracking toolbox, but perhaps the scale isn't going to be the best option for you. If you find that you are obsessing about the scale's movement (or lack thereof) and you start having overly diet-y thoughts after you weigh yourself, then put your scale away, smash it, or give it to someone you don't like. It's fine to be on team no-scale.

If you do want to use the scale and you fully understand and accept that body recomposition may skew your results, you absolutely must have a strategy that will help you mentally deal with your daily fluctuations. Otherwise, you may find yourself completely derailed by whatever number the scale shows you on a given morning. If the scale is up, you may say, *To heck with this!* and because you are frustrated with the number, you're tempted to eat all day. Your inner voice may say, *IF isn't working, so I may as well give up.* Or if the scale is down, your inner voice may tell you, *I'm doing great! Today I can have some treats because I am doing so well!*

Yep. Whether the scale is up *or* down, our inner voice can screw things up by popping in with diet-y thoughts in response to the number we see. So, what's an IFer to do?

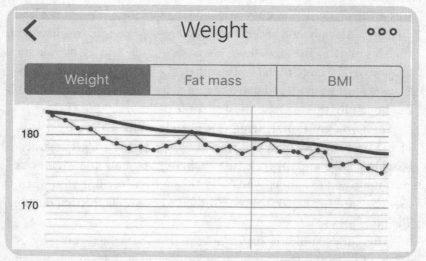

This is a photo of my weight graph from some point along the way in 2014. I had a scale that synced with my smartphone and the app created a graph of my progress.

I want to teach you something that will save your sanity and quiet your inner voice: the power of following your *overall weight trend only*.

On the previous page, I showed you a photo of my weight graph from some point along the way in 2014. I had a scale that synced with my smartphone and the app created a graph of my progress. Study that photo for a minute and pay attention to the two lines.

The jagged line shows my daily weights. Notice the pattern—my weight would go down for a few days and then it would spike back up for a few days, followed by some more downward movement and then another upward spike. The daily fluctuations could be quite frustrating! What was I doing wrong on the days when my weight went up? What was I doing *right* on the days when my weight went down? The answer to both questions is *nothing*; that's just what weight loss looks like. It won't be down, down, down, down, day after day. Unless you fully accept that fact, it's possible to make yourself crazy trying to understand your upward and downward swings.

Notice the solid line, however. That line shows my overall *trend*. Notice that the trend line has a gentle downward slope. *Only* the overall trend matters, and not the ups and downs.

The simplest way to track your trend is by using an app that does it for you like the one that came with my scale. My very favorite app is called Happy Scale, though there are others that do the same thing. These apps allow you to focus on the trend line, which should help you ignore the day-to-day fluctuations. If your overall trend line is going down, it is unimportant that today's weight may be higher. Never forget that weight fluctuates, and that is normal.

You may be more old-school, as I was. Even though I had the app that came with my scale, I wanted to have more data, and I enjoyed crunching the numbers myself. I also liked to compare my week-to-week progress, and I found that daily weighing with weekly averaging helped me fully understand what was going on with my overall trend.

I still have all the data from my weight-loss journey, and this is an actual sample of my daily weight record showing how I used weekly averaging. (If you look closely, you can find the weeks that go with

	SATURDAY	SUNDAY	MONDAY	TUESDAY	WEDNESDAY	THURSDAY	FRIDAY	WEEKLY AVERAGE	CHANGE
Row 1	185.1	184.2	184.9	185.2	185.3	185.0	185.1	185.0	—
Row 2	185.9	184.1	184.2	184.2	184.1	183.3	184.0	184.3	-0.7
Row 3	184.1	184.4	184.1	182.9	182.4	182.2	183.0	183.3	-1.0
Row 4	183.8	183.2	183.8	183.1	183.0	183.9	182.5	183.3	0
Row 5	183.6	183.2	183.0	183.4	182.4	181.9	182.8	182.9	-0.4
Row 6	182.5	183.2	182.5	181.9	180.8	180.7	179.3	181.6	-1.3
Row 7	178.7	178.0	178.2	177.8	178.4	178.9	180.3	178.6	-3.0
Row 8	178.6	177.8	178.4	177.4	178.1	179.3	177.7	178.2	-0.4
Row 9	177.7	176.9	177.9	175.8	175.9	176.4	175.4	176.6	-1.6
Row 10	174.7	176.6	176.6	177.3	176.5	175.2	176.3	176.2	-0.4
Row 11	176.6	177.9	177.0	174.7	172.5	170.9	169.6	174.2	-2.0

the weight graph that I shared; the data from the graph is found in rows 6–10.)

Notice all the fluctuations! My weight went up and down like crazy from day to day.

But! Notice my weekly averages. Most weeks, my weekly average was *down* (though there was that one week where it didn't go down at all, from row 3 to row 4). Some weeks it went down a lot (three pounds in row 7!), and some weeks it went down less than one pound. However, if you look at the *change* column and do the math, the *average change* was *exactly one pound per week,* even though some weeks the change was small and some weeks the change was large. Yep. Only the overall trend matters!

This is something for the ladies (men, if you want to skip this paragraph, go for it)—the days that are shaded darker are the weights I recorded during my menstrual cycle. Notice what happened in row 4: no weight loss at all. And then again in row 8: minimal weight loss. Over time, I understood that this was my body's pattern. No need to freak out or get upset; it's just what my body did. Getting upset wouldn't help, but understanding what was happening was powerful.

I want to use this data to illustrate another important point— infrequent weighing can be *worse* than never weighing. Yep. It's true. I do not recommend that you weigh once a week or once a month or whenever the spirit moves you. That is a recipe for a quick trip to Crazy-Town.

Let me explain.

What if I had only weighed myself on Fridays? In row 6, my Friday weight was 179.3. In row 7, my Friday weight was 180.3. When you look at the Friday-to-Friday weights, it looks like I gained a pound that week. But! If you look at the weekly averages, you can see that my weekly average for row 6 was 181.6, and my weekly average for row 7 was 178.6. It's true! My greatest average weekly change just so happened to occur on a week where my Friday-to-Friday weight was *up*. Instead of being discouraged by a pound "gain," I knew that I was down an *average* of *three pounds*. Hooray for weekly averaging!

If I only weighed occasionally, that would also be a problem. If I weighed on the Tuesday of row 9 (175.8) and then again on the Sunday of row 11 (177.9) I would think I had gained *over two pounds*! That would be really discouraging! When I look at my weekly averages, however, I see that my weekly average for row 9 was 176.6, and my weekly average for row 11 was 174.2. My weekly average was down by over two pounds!

If you want to calculate your weekly average manually as I did but you can't remember how to do it, it's time for a math lesson. We find the weekly average by adding up all the numbers for the week (you should have 7 numbers), and then dividing the sum by 7.

Let's illustrate how this works using the numbers from row 1:

$$185.1 + 184.2 + 184.9 + 185.2 + 185.3 + 185.0 + 185.1 = 1,294.8$$
$$1,294.8 \div 7 = \mathbf{185.0}$$

(It was actually 184.971429, but I rounded it to the nearest tenth.)

If you hate math and this example makes you think back to your school days and tremble with fear, get an app. It's perfectly fine. (Remember how our teachers told us that we wouldn't always have a calculator with us, so we needed to know how to do this stuff by hand? Good times. And we showed them, didn't we? Thanks, smartphones!)

Another weighing strategy that works well for some is even more old-school, but it's absolutely genius for people who can't stand seeing the upward fluctuations at all and *only* want to see the downward trend. For this method, get yourself an old-fashioned balance scale like the ones they might have in a doctor's office, and tell everyone in your family that they aren't allowed to touch it. When you weigh the first time, slide it to reflect your weight that day, and then step off. The next day, get on it again. This is the important part: *only* adjust the number if you need to adjust it downward! If your weight is up, and the scale no longer balances, get off and go about your day as if nothing happened *without adjusting the number*. You get to ignore the fluctuation entirely, and because you didn't even slide the bar over, it's like it doesn't exist. Over time, you'll get to slowly adjust the scale to lower and lower numbers, but you never have to see the numbers reflected in the upward spikes.

I hope that I have convinced you of the importance of weighing regularly and understanding what your overall trend is doing rather than getting caught up in the madness of fluctuating weights. I believe that most of the people who start IF but give up quit because they are allowing daily fluctuations to both rule the day and to convince them that IF isn't working. Either have a daily weighing strategy for noting your overall trend or get rid of the scale entirely. It's that important.

Now that you understand how to use the scale as a tool for tracking your progress, let's move on to the next strategy: measuring!

On day 0 and again on day 29, you took these measurements:

Measurements:
Bust or chest: _____
Waist: _____
Hips: _____
Right thigh: _____
Left thigh: _____

As I mentioned to you in the FAST Start chapter, you can track other areas as well if you would like to. If you are not sure about *how* to measure yourself accurately, do a Google search or find an instructional video on YouTube that shows you proper measuring technique.

The key is that you are going to measure yourself in the same areas, using the same techniques, once every two weeks or so, and see how the various areas of your body are changing. Expect to see slow and yet steady changes over time.

One of the most important measurements to focus on is your waist, and honestly, if you only want to measure *one* place, this is the one to measure, since our waist sizes are linked to so many health outcomes (in study after study, we find that a smaller waist = positive health outcomes, and a larger waist = negative health outcomes). While I don't weigh anymore, I *do* measure my waist from time to time, and it helps me to know that I am weight-stable.

If you really want to get scientific and math-y, you can track something known as your *waist-to-height ratio*. To do this, you can use an online calculator, or you can do some math: take your waist measurement and divide it by your height measurement. Why does it matter? Science shows us that the waist-to-height ratio is a better predictor of mortality risk (meaning *death*) than BMI.[1] A higher value also indicates a higher risk of obesity-related illnesses. A waist-to-height ratio below 0.5 is healthier, while a 0.57 and above puts you into the obese range.

Just for fun, I calculated mine. My waist-to-height ratio is 0.415, and when I asked Uncle Google for a table of waist-to-height comparisons, I found that I fall right between a female college swimmer (0.42) and Beyoncé (0.38). I also noted that my waist-to-height ratio puts me in the "slim" category. Not too shabby for a formerly obese fifty-year-old woman who doesn't swim *or* go on world tour!

One other important ratio you may want to consider keeping tabs on is your waist-to-hip ratio. As with the waist-to-height ratio, this is a better marker of health than BMI. A lower waist-to-hip ratio is linked to lower levels of cardiovascular disease and diabetes and also to increased fertility.[2] You can find an online calculator or do the math yourself; take your waist measurement and divide it by your hip measurement.

I calculated my own waist-to-hip ratio and got a 0.69. According to one source, a 0.70 is "ideal" for female fertility, and even though I am *way* past my childbearing years, I was happy to find that I have a "fertile figure." One chart I saw indicated that my ratio puts me in the "pear shaped" category, which is no surprise.

Besides using the scale and measurements, a third valuable tool for measuring progress is the practice of comparing photos of yourself. When using this strategy, make sure to take photos of yourself from the front, from the side, and from the back. If possible, get someone else to take them for you, but mirror selfies also work.

If you are taking progress photos (and I really hope that you do, because I think this is the most powerful strategy of all), make sure that you wear the exact same clothes every time! You can study how the clothes fit in the photos and really see the changes in your body. I remember taking a photo of myself wearing my favorite dress after I had lost about twenty-five pounds. I re-created the older photo exactly: I stood in the same place, I put on the same jewelry, and I tried to hold my arms in the same position. When I compared the two photos, I really could see how much my body had changed. Heck, I could see that even my necklace hung farther down on my neck, as apparently I even had a chubby neck in the earlier photo!

Also, even though you are taking these photos for your own viewing pleasure *now*, I recommend that you wear either real clothes or a swimsuit. Why? When you have stunning success, you are going to want to show these photos to other people. And if you took photos in your underwear or while naked, you really should keep those to yourself, #AmIRight? You'll thank yourself later for having PG photos that show your progress and that you can also share with your friends and family members. Grandma doesn't want to see you in your undies.

Finally, I want to introduce you to the final tool in your measurement toolbox: honesty pants. For this strategy, you will have one article of clothing in the next size (or two) down to use as a goal. I like to use a pair of pants that have absolutely no stretch to them at all, because that's going to give me the best feedback. Every week or two, try the pants on for size, and over time, notice how the fit changes . . . until one day, BOOM! The pants fit! What to do next? You guessed it! Get a new pair of honesty pants and repeat the process. Even if the scale isn't moving, always trust your honesty pants.

Now that I have taught you about all the tools to keep in your measurement toolbox, I have one other thing I want to talk about, and it's the most important concept of all.

This is *so important* to understand, y'all.

If *something* is changing, *you are making progress!*

Here is what I mean by that:

- If the scale is trending downward slowly over time (on your app or when looking at your weekly averages), *you are making progress,* no matter what your measurements or photos show!

- If your measurements are going downward slowly over time, *you are making progress,* no matter what the scale says or your photos show!

- If you look slimmer in your photos, *you are making progress,* no matter what the scale or tape measure show!

- If your honesty pants fit, *you are making progress,* no matter what the scale, tape measure, or photos tell you!

So many people make the mistake of fixating on the measurements that are *not* changing and ignoring the ones that are! Don't let that happen to you. If *something* is changing, it's working!

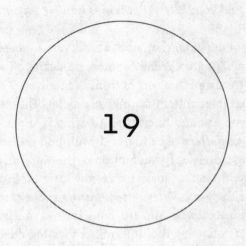

19

LIFESTYLE VERSUS DIET: THERE IS NO WAGON

How many times have you started a new diet and soon began longing for the day when you would reach your goal weight and could stop the madness and return to your old ways of eating? Or how many times did you take a weekend off (or a week, or a month, or a year . . .) and then realized you had "fallen off the wagon" completely?

Yep. Me, too. *So many times.* In fact, I did that with every single diet I ever tried. Sooner or later (usually sooner), I would abandon the plan entirely and move on to something else (which usually included a rebound phase where I ate like a teenage boy going through a growth spurt in direct response to the over-restriction of whatever "diet" I had been on, which is exactly what we know happens when our bodies crank up our hunger hormones in response to over-restriction).

The good news is that intermittent fasting is completely different.

What if I told you: **With IF,** *there is no diet wagon,* **so you can't "fall off it."**

Once you understand that, now, at this very moment of your life, you can take a big sigh of relief. No more on-again, off-again diets for you! You are *free* from that sort of thinking forever.

Realize that intermittent fasting *isn't* a diet. The word *diet* refers to the foods you eat, and intermittent fasting is about *when* you eat, not what. IF is a *pattern* of eating, and your food choices fit within it.

So, looking closely at the definition of the word *diet,* you can see that intermittent fasting doesn't meet the criteria. Promise me you will never use the words *intermittent fasting* and *diet* together to describe what you are doing. You are living the intermittent fasting *lifestyle,* and NOT following the "intermittent fasting diet."

So, is intermittent fasting really a lifestyle that you can follow forever? The answer is a resounding YES.

Recently, I conducted a survey of members in one of my online IF support groups asking how they felt about intermittent fasting. While this is not a scientific survey (and I don't claim that it is), a full 99.9 percent of respondents said that intermittent fasting is their "forever lifestyle."

I asked, "What do you think about intermittent fasting?" The choices were:

1. IF is my forever lifestyle.

2. IF is a temporary diet, and I'll stop when I get to my goal weight.

3. Who am I, and why am I here?

Yes, I added that third option as a joke, because I wanted to lighten up the moment.

Eight hours after posting the survey, more than 1,200 group members had chosen "IF is my forever lifestyle," while only 3 people selected the option "IF is a temporary diet, and I'll stop when I get to my goal weight." Yes. Only 3 people, versus over 1,200 who viewed IF as their forever lifestyle. (Funny story—15 people selected option C. Those are my favorite people, the jokesters of the world. I probably would have picked that one, too. Bless.)

WOW! I knew intermittent fasters were committed, but these results surprised even me! I dare you to ask that question in any other "diet" group! (I put "diet" in quotation marks, because remember . . . IF is NOT a diet!) Most people can't *wait* to stop a diet and get back to "real life." That's clearly not true for IFers! As I said, this is clearly not a scientific survey that follows rigorous survey design (not even close), but it was still eye-opening. *More people selected the joke answer* than picked the option that IF was something they were doing only until reaching their goal weight. That is powerful insight. #LifestyleNotDiet.

Remember that intermittent fasting is the health plan with a side effect of weight loss, so there is no reason why you would ever *want* to stop living the intermittent fasting lifestyle! Most long-term IFers realize that they never want to stop living an IF lifestyle because of how great they feel, and that's exactly what I bet you'll discover.

If you're new to IF and striving to make it feel like a true lifestyle for you, you may need some tools to help you cement intermittent fasting as a habit. One tool that works well for many is a fasting app.

People like to joke about using a fasting app, and they'll say something like, "My fasting app is a clock, and I just look at that." Nothing wrong with keeping it simple! I don't use a fasting app, either. Well, I don't *now*.

Back in 2016, however, I found an app to be very handy. I was a year into maintenance and still experimenting with fasting styles. I had also just discovered the clean fast, which made a huge difference in the way I experienced my daily fast. During the spring of 2016, I had been experimenting with 4:3, and it worked well for my body, but I decided that I wanted to switch to a daily eating window long term. I knew that I wanted to track my eating-window length on an app, but I couldn't find one that allowed me to customize my eating window; all the apps that were out at that time only allowed you to track your fast. My son is a computer programmer and app developer, and he just happened to be home from college, so I asked him to make an app for me. He did, and I started using it.

Using that app really helped me cement the daily-eating-window habit. I used it daily for months, and it was psychologically pleasing to "close my window" on the app. Once I did that, I was a lot less likely to pop something into my mouth . . . nope! My window was closed!

Funny story. I made it a goal of mine to have a "perfect" month; I would have an entire month where my eating window never went beyond five hours! May of 2016? Nope. June of 2016? Nope. July? August? September? Nope, nope, and nope. I *never* had a perfect month, based on my goal of keeping my eating window to five hours or less every single day. And guess what? It didn't even matter! During that time, even though I was in maintenance and not trying to lose any more weight, I lost one full size in jeans. I also wasn't weighing myself, and that was freeing in and of itself. So, learn from my experience. You won't be perfect, and I certainly wasn't, even when I set perfection as my goal. Perfection is overrated, anyway; I chose brunch instead. And that was even more perfect, in my opinion.

When October rolled around, I realized that I didn't even *need* the app anymore. My IF eating window was fully on autopilot! Every day, I opened my window, I ate, I stopped when satisfied, and my window closed whenever it closed. The freedom was remarkable! From that point on, I have never again tracked my eating window closely. I still get in a daily fast, and most days, my eating window is five hours or less, but not every day. I find that it balances out; one day my window might be longer, and the next day it seems to be naturally shorter. I think this is part of appetite correction for me, actually.

Now there are lots of apps available to you, and you can choose to track your eating window, track your fast, or even join a fasting circle to meet other IFers who are fasting right along with you! Browse through the app stores available for your device and see which look appealing to you. Use the apps until your own IF protocol is on autopilot, or use it because you love data! Or don't use one at all. It's totally up to you.

Even so, understand that you will have days with longer eating windows and shorter fasts, and that's just part of life. When I went to my son's college graduation, I didn't "fall off the wagon" when I decided to open my window with a delicious brunch at 10:00 a.m.—I embraced the idea that on that particular day, my fast was shorter. On my fiftieth birthday, I didn't even hesitate when I opened my eating window at midday with cocktails and snacks on the beach with friends. On both occasions, I made a choice, and I made it with zero guilt. When you decide to have a day with a longer eating window, you aren't "cheating," and you haven't ruined anything! So, there are no diet sins to atone for. That's diet mentality, and remember that IF isn't a diet.

When you begin your IF lifestyle, however, you won't want to throw caution to the winds anytime the mood strikes you. During the FAST Start, you are building up your fasting muscle, and consistency is what helps your body deplete glycogen stores so you can ignite your fat-burning superpower. I recommend *not* allowing yourself to be too flexible with your schedule during the FAST Start or it will take you longer to get through the adjustment phase and make it harder for you in the long run.

Even when you're an experienced IFer, you still want to remain consistent with your fasting most of the time; if you have too many long eating windows and short fasts, you'll keep your glycogen stores fully stocked and your body won't *need* to tap into fat stores at all! Always remember why we are fasting!

When you go on a vacation, you may be worried about how IF will fit into your life. The good news is that vacations are a lot easier as an IFer than they were before IF!

One of my favorite vacations is to go on a cruise. Before IF, I would view the entire trip as a free-for-all, and the "diet" would start once I got back. (Actually, the "diet" usually started a couple of weeks before I left, when I realized that my body wasn't swimsuit ready. That never helped, though.)

You probably think of cruises as nothing but days and days of pure gluttony, and that is how I used to view a cruise. I would be the first one in line for breakfast, I always ate a full lunch, and then every night was a sit-down dinner, not to mention the late-night snacks! My "Help! I'm obese and I'm miserable!" wake-up call actually came to me on a family cruise in 2014; I weighed 210 pounds, and the photos of us showed me the truth: I was full, sick, and miserable, and when I looked at those photos, I vowed that this was going to be the last time I felt that way. I came back from that cruise and took control of my life, and everything is different.

Now? I no longer view a vacation as a free-for-all because I don't like the way I *feel* when I overeat. When we are packed and ready to go, I get into the car in the fasted state, and I spend the entire drive to the port in the fasted state, as well. It's a lot more enjoyable than traveling while loaded up on junk food or fast food. I'm such a food snob now that none of that road food is very appealing, unlike before.

When I step onto the cruise ship, my window is open! I start with a fruity cocktail or glass of champagne and some sort of snack. I don't want to ruin my appetite for the sit-down dinner in the main dining room. When dinner rolls around, I frequently choose a vegetarian option, because I have learned two things: first of all, the vegetarian options are usually some of the best meals on any cruise ship, and second, I am less likely to find myself overly full when I stick to high-quality foods, even on a cruise ship. Dessert? Don't mind if I do! I may choose a chocolate dessert, some cheesecake, or even a fruit-and-cheese plate.

During the other days of the cruise, I focus on eating mindfully. I usually skip breakfast, although I might have brunch once or twice if I feel like it. Usually my eating windows are anywhere from eight to twelve hours every day, and I play it by ear. My goal is to never feel overly full, and rather than tightly controlling my eating window length, I focus on stopping when satisfied.

When it's time to disembark, I start fasting, and I fast all the way home. My body is so ready for a fast! It feels wonderful to get back to normal. For a few days after returning home, I'm usually tired and draggy. Biologically, it's easy to understand why! On the cruise, I ate a lot more food than usual, and I refilled my glycogen stores. It takes a few days of my normal routine to deplete those glycogen stores again, and so I might need a nap in the afternoon for a few days. Soon, though, I'm back to normal.

Again, keep in mind that I didn't fall off the wagon or cheat while on my cruise. I chose to have longer windows and shorter fasts, and I enjoyed every moment with no guilt. I didn't have to do longer fasts when I got back home to make up for the trip, either. All I had to do is resume my regular IF protocol, and it was all good.

If you are someone who weighs, keep in mind that after a vacation, your weight is likely to be up by a *lot*. One time (back when I used to weigh daily), I "gained" *nine pounds* after a particularly luxurious girls' trip. I didn't freak out; I simply went back to my preferred IF routine. By the following weekend, I was back to normal. Remember that not only does food weigh a lot, but you'll retain a lot of fluid along with the food. It's not all fat gain!

This is what I want you to take away from this chapter: You're not on a diet, and so you don't need to have words like *diet, falling off the wagon,* or *cheating* in your vocabulary any longer. You can lose the guilt, enjoy special occasions and vacations, and know that IF is either there with you making the occasion or trip more enjoyable or at least waiting for you when you get back home.

We fast.

We feast . . . *sometimes more than other times!*

We repeat.

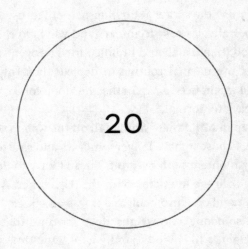

20

GET YOUR MIND RIGHT!

Confession: intermittent fasting didn't work for me.

Until it did.

I first learned about intermittent fasting in 2009. I can't remember which book I read first, but I know there were several that served as my introduction to fasting as a weight-loss tool (because that is *all* I considered IF to be at that time: a method to use for weight loss). There wasn't much to choose from back then; I read Dr. Bert Herring's first book, *The Fast-5 Diet and the Fast-5 Lifestyle,* Brad Pilon's ebook, *Eat. Stop. Eat.,* and two books about the up-and-down-day approach, Dr. John Daugirdas's *The QOD Diet* (*QOD* means *every other day*) and Dr. James Johnson's *The Alternate-Day Diet* (2008 version).

All these books piqued my interest because it seemed so simple to have a daily eating window (*Fast-5*) or to take a twenty-four-hour break from eating a few times per week (*Eat. Stop. Eat.*). I also loved the idea of dieting only every other day (*QOD* and *Alternate-Day*

Diet). It certainly seemed a lot simpler than trying to diet all day, every day. Now, *that* was hard!

Even though I instinctively knew at that time that intermittent fasting was going to be my long-term answer, I was a mess. Yep. A complete failure.

Looking back, it really is mind-boggling to me to view my stunning failure, since I'm someone who eventually lost over eighty pounds and has gone on to maintain the loss effortlessly for years now. It's ironic that *I had the secret right there in my hands, and I failed and failed and failed*. From 2009 to 2014, I guess I would call myself an IF "dabbler." I would try Fast-5 for a couple of weeks. Then I would stop completely. Next, I would try a week of up-and-down days, until something came up and I would abandon it all. Or I would have so many up days in a row that I would forget to even try having a down day. Maybe I would decide to follow *Eat. Stop. Eat.* and have a twenty-four-hour fast, but something always came up that would mean I broke my fast before getting to the twenty-four-hour mark.

There were several things that held me back:

- I was not fasting clean.

- Results were not quick or linear.

- I never gave it enough time to allow my body to adapt to fasting.

- I had a dieter's mind-set.

Let's look at each of those one by one and see how they kept me from being successful during those years.

First, I was not fasting clean. Heck, the phrase *fasting clean* hadn't even been coined yet. In the early days of my IF journey, I thought that fasting only worked because it allowed us to eat fewer calories. If you are following the "only calories matter when trying to lose weight" paradigm, then you would think diet sodas, gum, coffee creamer, and so on couldn't possibly make a difference in your weight loss. (Now, we totally understand why that is false, as I explained in the clean fast chapters.) As a result of not fasting clean, I was constantly starving, and every minute of the fast, I was white-knuckling it until it was time to eat. No wonder I kept stopping! Fasting was *hard*.

Next, results were not quick enough for me. I may have been weighing daily, but I had completely unrealistic expectations. (I'm not sure if you have seen the meme: "I don't always diet, but when I do, I expect the results to be instant, dramatic, and spectacular," but that concept *totally* applied to me back then.) Every day, I would get on the scale. And every day, I expected the scale to show a lower number than it had the day before. As I discussed in a previous chapter, weight loss is not linear, and our bodies can fluctuate a great deal from day to day. Mine sure did. On those days when my scale was up, that was all I needed to convince myself that fasting wasn't working, and I would quit in disgust.

Because I kept starting and quitting and starting and quitting, I never gave my body a chance to adapt to fasting. As I mentioned in the 28-Day FAST Start chapter, the adjustment phase is the most difficult part of fasting, and I never made it out of the adjustment phase. Basically, I lived in the adjustment phase. Sigh. Couple that with the fact that I wasn't fasting clean, and I was doomed to failure.

Finally, I had a total dieter's mind-set. I had it in my head that dieting was something you did short term, it should work quickly, and then you were able to go back to "normal" and you would magically stay slim forever. Problem solved! Except that isn't at all how it works, is it? When you are trapped in dieter's mind-set, you are always either "on" the diet or "off" the diet. (And this is a good time to remind you that intermittent fasting is a lifestyle, not a diet. Remember that you will *never* see me use the words *intermittent fasting* and *diet* together, and you shouldn't, either. You are not on the "intermittent fasting diet." You are living the intermittent fasting lifestyle. The difference may seem subtle, but it is *huge*.)

Because I had a dieter's mind-set, I also let my inner toddler take over. *I want it NOW!* I could always fast tomorrow, which is just like the dieter who always plans to start again on Monday. I would sit looking wistfully at the people eating around me ALL. DAY. LONG. I smelled their delicious lunches. (Funny how a frozen diet meal can suddenly look appealing.) I saw them drinking their coffees with fancy flavored creamer, and I resented that *they* "got to" eat, drink, and be merry, while I was sitting there counting the hours until I could break my fast.

The good news is that *you* are not going to make the same mistakes I made. You understand the importance of fasting clean. (If not, go back and reread that chapter. Go ahead. I'll wait. It's that important.) You understand that results aren't going to be quick, and they aren't going to be linear; the scale won't go down, down, down, day after day, and there will be both upward fluctuations and plateaus along the way. You also understand that it's important to give your body time to adjust to fasting, and you have the 28-Day FAST Start to cement the clean fast as your habit.

The final piece of the puzzle will be getting your **mind** in the right place. So, let's take some time to learn about why mind-set is so important and how making simple shifts in your thought processes can make all the difference between success and failure for you.

The right mind-set can change your whole life.

No, this is not hippie-dippie talk. There is actual science behind these concepts, and it's more important than you think!

There's a powerful quote that's attributed to Henry Ford:

> Whether you think you can or you think you can't, you're right.

We have all heard this quote before, haven't we? You may think it sounds overly simple or like wishful thinking, but I'm going to teach you the science behind it, and it's completely fascinating.

As you know, I was an elementary teacher, and I spent twenty-eight years in the classroom. One of the most important books I ever read was a book called *Mindset,* written by Dr. Carol Dweck. The book is based on Dr. Dweck's research into the importance of a person's mind-set. As an example, she found that when children feel like their success is related to hard work and perseverance, which she calls a "growth mindset," they are willing to take on challenges and persevere through difficulties. If, however, they are trapped in a "fixed mindset," they feel like their abilities are "fixed," and therefore they are unwilling to take risks or push through certain challenges. Based on her research, I completely changed the way I spoke to children, and I found that it made a tremendous difference in my classroom. I no longer told children they were "smart" or that they were "good at" something. Instead, I mentioned how hard they had worked to master a skill or asked them to explain how they figured something out. When they were having trouble with something, I asked them to try to figure out why they were having that particular issue and then encouraged them to make a plan to overcome the challenge.

Because of this change, I found that my students were more willing to take risks, and they were also willing to fail. The goal was for the kids to understand that it takes hard work to do anything worthwhile, and while everyone has certain strengths and weaknesses, we are not stuck with our current abilities.

Anything worth doing takes work (including intermittent fasting), and we are all capable of growth. If you are interested in learning more about the research related to mind-set, I can't recommend Dr. Dweck's book highly enough, and if you have kids in your life who are important to you, then you can apply her research to the way you speak to them. I believe that it makes a huge difference long term.

I have applied this research on the importance of mind-set into my personal life, as well. We can get stuck in certain types of thinking that affect our lives in many ways. For example, I mentioned that I used to be trapped in a diet mind-set. I felt like I was either on a diet or I was off it. I was either being "good" on my diet, or I was "cheating." And so I was always either losing weight or I was gaining weight, depending on whether I was "on" or "off"; "good" or "bad." Can you relate to that? If you have as much dieting history as I do, I am sure you can.

As I said, when I first discovered intermittent fasting, I approached it with my typical diet mind-set. I thought I would follow it until I got to my goal, and then I would figure out how to maintain my loss in a way that allowed me to "eat like a normal person" as much as possible. I viewed intermittent fasting as a temporary fix to a temporary problem. What I didn't realize is that the diet mind-set was my *permanent* problem, and that was the thing I needed to fix. And I needed to fix it *permanently.* Only by losing the diet mind-set could I finally lose the weight I also needed to lose. When I realized that intermittent fasting needed to be my *lifestyle* to maintain the eighty-plus-pound loss, it made a tremendous difference. I wasn't going to stop intermittent fasting, and there was no end point at which time I could declare I was done. I had officially conquered the diet mind-set, and it felt great. Now I am confident that I will *never* "diet" again!

For a long part of the process, I was also stuck in the "can't" mind-set. I "can't" eat until 5:00. I "can't" eat when everyone else is eating. I "can't" put delicious creamers in my coffee. I was focused on deprivation, which is a carryover of my old diet mind-set. Instead of enjoying the fasting time, I put my attention onto what I couldn't do. I have to admit—sometimes, fasting during the day felt like torture that I had to tolerate until it was time to eat. I saw coworkers, friends, or family members eating breakfast and lunch, and I felt disgruntled. Why couldn't I eat like everyone else? I deserved it!

This is so important! If you're still stuck in the "can't" mind-set, it's time to change that. You will *never* enjoy the intermittent fasting lifestyle until you get rid of the "can't" mentality.

One of the keys to my success is that I have completely changed my self-talk. I no longer tell myself that I "deserve" to eat just because everyone else is eating. No, I tell myself that I deserve to be slim and healthy! Once I made that particular mind shift, I could watch others eat without feeling the least bit disgruntled. I can cook breakfast for my family and not even have one moment where I feel like I should be eating along with them. Whenever you start to feel like you deserve to eat something, remember that what you really deserve is to be healthy.

What about the "can't" mind-set? How do you conquer that particular feeling? Recall all the amazing benefits of an intermittent fasting lifestyle, and remember—it's not all about weight loss (though we aren't mad about that particular benefit, are we?). No, it's about having vibrant health! You have discovered the fountain of youth! To remind yourself of some of these amazing health benefits, reread chapters 2 and 3 about the health and longevity benefits of intermittent fasting whenever you need a pep talk.

Embrace the fast itself. Instead of thinking of the fast as something you have to get through so you can get to your eating window, spend some time each day valuing the time you spend in the fasted state. Recognize that the fast is when your body is focused on healing and repair. Appreciate the sustained energy and mental clarity you feel while fasting. Never forget that the magic happens in the clean fast! Once you make these important mental shifts, you learn to appreciate the fasting time every bit as much as you appreciate the delicious foods that you eat in your eating window.

It's not that you *can't* eat frequently; it's that you *choose not to*! After learning about intermittent fasting, you now know it's better for your body to not be constantly in the fed state. You are *choosing* to give your body a long period each day to take care of cellular housekeeping; one side effect happens to be that you will eventually lose your excess fat and then you'll be at your ideal weight forever. WIN-WIN, PEOPLE! Where's the deprivation there? I certainly didn't feel deprived when I bought my first pair of size 0 jeans (though I was pretty incredulous; thank you, vanity sizing). When you view fasting through the lens of health and longevity, you realize that you are only depriving yourself of the diseases related to the overconsumption of food and constant insulin release. I am excited to deprive myself of those health problems!

Another thing that really helps me keep my mind right is thinking about my future self. No, not my years-from-now future self but my future self who lives one hour in the future. When I have the thought that I would like to open my window early, I think about how I will feel in one hour. In one hour, will I be glad that I ate whatever looks appealing now, or will I feel regretful? If I know I will be glad to have participated in that particular eating experience, I open my window without a backward glance and embrace the moment without a twinge of guilt. If I know I will be sorry later that I did it, I don't eat. This little technique is very helpful for me, and it's the *delay* in action! Eating earlier in the day makes me feel lethargic, and I lose the awesome mental clarity that I enjoy while in the fasted state. It absolutely has to be worth it for me to give that up!

Oh, and understand that my personal mental shifts didn't happen overnight. Give it time. Most important, work on changing your self-talk so that you can shift your mind-set for good. I promise that life is better on the other side!

Earlier in this chapter, I promised that I would explain some of the science behind the very real power of our beliefs, and I have saved some of the best for last. Before I share it with you, I want you to take a few minutes to contemplate these questions and your answers to them:

- Right this minute, do you *believe* that intermittent fasting will work for you?

- Do you *truly* believe in the health benefits of IF?

- Do you believe that *you* can experience the weight loss that you are hoping for?

Belief is powerful.

If you don't believe that intermittent fasting will work for you or you think you're a hopeless case and you will never lose weight, then *those very thoughts* are likely holding you back.

You have to *believe* that your body is equipped to tap into your stored fat for fuel. You have to *believe* that whatever has held you back before is in the past, and now you are doing something new and powerful. You have to *believe* that your body is capable of supporting vibrant health.

I'm not talking about "Believe you can have a Cadillac and before you know it, you'll have a Cadillac in your driveway!" We aren't wishing for things like you'd wish for presents from Santa Claus.

Have you heard of the placebo effect? This phenomenon is when people experience a measurable benefit to a drug or a treatment that they *think* they are receiving, even though they have not received an actual drug or treatment. The placebo is usually something like a sugar pill or a fake "treatment" instead of the real thing. It turns out that the expectations of the patient are key; the more a person expects the treatment to work, the more likely it is to work, even if they receive a placebo!

How does the placebo effect work? This is still a matter of debate. In a 2016 study, scientists found that participants who experienced pain relief after taking a placebo had greater activity in the frontal lobes of their brains.[1] This isn't just wishing away the pain; this is evidence for a biological response to the placebo! The patients *believed* they would have pain relief, a certain part of their brain had a biological response to the treatment, and they reported less pain.

I have always been fascinated with this topic! Here are three studies that are particularly interesting:

- Eighty-four female hotel workers were split into two groups. One group was told that the work they do cleaning hotel rooms was great exercise and met all recommendations for an active lifestyle, and the other group was not given this information. Four weeks later, the group who believed they were getting all the exercise they needed through their work had significant decreases in weight, blood pressure, body fat, waist-to-hip ratio, and BMI, and the other group did not have these positive changes.[2]

- Ninety participants with a normal weight were split into three groups who all received the same placebo, but one group was told that the drug would increase appetite, the second group was told it should increase satiety, and the third group was told the drug would not affect appetite either way. Not only is this what happened in every single group (what they were *told* would happen is what *happened*), but the group who believed they would have an increased appetite had a measurable *increase* in their *levels of ghrelin,* the hunger hormone. Yep! There was an actual biological response that the scientists could measure![3]

- Fourteen healthy yet overweight adults were split into two groups. Each group was given the exact same diet, with a number of calories designed to keep the participants at a stable weight. One group was told they were following a low-calorie diet that would result in a weight loss of about 6 kg in eight weeks, and the other group was told that it was a diet designed to keep them at their current weights. The group who *believed* they were on a low-calorie regimen lost an average of 9.25 kg, or 20 pounds, within that eight-week period! The other group also lost weight, but only about 2.25 kg, or about 5 pounds. They followed the same diet, but the group who *believed* they would lose weight lost *four times more weight.*[4]

Wowza. I love this stuff, y'all.

In addition to the placebo effect, we have other studies that illustrate the power of the mind:

- Participants who *imagined* they were doing physical activity had *improved muscle strength,* even though they were only doing the physical activity in their minds![5]

- Those with a positive self-perception of aging lived *7.5 years longer* than those with a more negative perception of aging.[6]

- In a thirty-year study, optimists were found to have better physical and mental health outcomes, and those identified as pessimists had a 19 percent higher mortality rate.[7,8] Optimists were also found to have significantly better cardiovascular health markers.[9]

These are just a few of the many studies that are out there, but I hope you are convinced that mind-set matters. As you can see, the mind is a powerful thing!

How can you apply this information about mind-set and belief to your intermittent fasting practice?

I would like to give you a mind-set and belief action plan that you can use to help you make the mental shifts you need.

- Study the health benefits of intermittent fasting until you understand how powerful IF can be. This gives you confidence that what you are doing is healthy for your body.

- Understand *how* IF allows you to tap into your fat stores, and know that *your* body can do it, too! The fat is stored on your body to fuel you, and when you give your body time to access it, you'll turn on your natural fat-burning superpower.

- Remain optimistic that you will be able to figure out just the right IF protocol for your body, and that you *can* tweak it till it's easy!

- If you find yourself slipping into self-doubt, reread the chapters of this book that speak to your specific concerns or struggle.

- Surround yourself with positive people, and find a support system that is full of other intermittent fasters. Community is powerful!

- Embrace the power of the fast and celebrate that time of your life just as much as you enjoy the feast. Both are an essential part of your intermittent fasting practice!

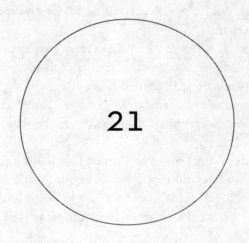

21

GET MOVING!
FAST-FUELED FITNESS

Many new (and even experienced) intermittent fasters have questions about exercise, so let's take some time to tackle the most common questions and concerns. Before we do, though, I need to get one thing out of the way. If you are an endurance athlete or a serious bodybuilder, you're going to need more guidance than I can give you in one chapter. Also, you are going to need more guidance than I am *qualified* to give you! I prefer to build muscles by hauling around cases of San Pellegrino, and my favorite cardio workout is Hula-Hooping. So, for specific protocols that would suit a more intense exercise regimen, look for a source that understands the science of intermittent fasting and can help you reach your fitness goals. There are both bodybuilders and endurance athletes out there who are achieving amazing results by strategically incorporating intermittent fasting into their training protocols. I'll touch on some of the science here in this chapter, but for practical training advice and specifics, you'll need to dig deeper.

The good news is that if you're an average person or even a more casual fitness enthusiast, this chapter will probably answer most of your questions related to IF and exercise.

First, is exercise required for weight loss? No. Exercise alone is unlikely to result in meaningful or significant weight loss, and studies have backed this up.[1]

Now, before you get upset and think I am telling you *not* to exercise, please understand that I am saying nothing of the sort. Exercise is essential for overall health and well-being and is linked to many positive physical and mental outcomes, as well as increased longevity.[2]

We have enough evidence to say with confidence that regular physical exercise helps us prevent chronic diseases, such as diabetes, cancer, osteoporosis, and cardiovascular disease, just to name a few.[3] We also know that lack of exercise and poor overall fitness is a strong predictor of early death. And routine physical activity is associated with a reduction of stress, anxiety, and depression.[4]

So, YES. Exercise is an essential part of a healthy lifestyle.

Now you may wonder: What is the best type of exercise to do? People ask this all the time, and I have the definitive answer that you have been waiting for! Based on all my years of research . . .

Drumroll, please!

The best type of exercise for you to do is . . . **Any type of exercise you enjoy and that you will do regularly!**

Sorry, was that anticlimactic? Were you expecting me to extoll the virtues of cardio or wax poetic about the importance of resistance training?

All joking aside, I think we need to do both; we need to move our bodies in ways that promote excellent cardiovascular health, and we also need to do things that require us to work our muscles.

There are so many ways you can accomplish these goals, though! Yes, structured fitness classes and gym memberships are one way to go. Or you can try to be more active and less sedentary as you live your life. You may think there is no benefit to these more casual activities, but you would be incorrect![5,6] In one study, just thirty minutes of light activity each day was linked to a lower risk of death, and an even greater benefit was found from the addition of moderate-intensity exercise. Things you already do—running errands, vacuuming the house, cooking dinner, and mowing the lawn—absolutely count as light activity! And taking a walk around your neighborhood or riding your bike can be fun ways to get in more moderate-intensity exercise. No gym membership or fancy workout clothes required—just get up off the couch and get moving!

As I mentioned in the beginning of this chapter, I'm not someone who enjoys a structured exercise regimen. I *do,* however, enjoy feeling strong and nimble on my feet. I look at my arms and see great muscle definition, which I achieved by carrying heavy things or scrubbing the bathtub. I can walk along the beach for hours and play in the surf. One day, I'll run around with my grandchildren. I want to be the centenarian who can jog circles around those youngsters in their seventies and eighties, so I plan to always keep moving as I age.

There is one other factor when deciding which exercise might be right for you: genetics! We have learned that our bodies are different when it comes to what foods work well for us, and while many of these differences are related to our gut microbiomes, some are also related to our DNA. Just as scientists can use algorithms to predict our ideal foods, they have been able to develop algorithms to match our genotypes to our ideal training protocols.[7] When participants were matched with their ideal programs, they saw significant improvements in both power-based and endurance-based activities.

As you know, I had my DNA analyzed, and the results confirmed a lot of what I'd already suspected. No, my report didn't say I should take up Hula-Hooping specifically, but there were other findings that matched what I already knew. As an example, my report lists me as someone who "may not experience much weight loss" with exercise. That probably explains why I *never* have experienced increased weight loss related to an exercise regimen. You, however, may be in the "likely to experience higher weight loss" category, so perhaps you think I'm crazy when I tell you exercise isn't a part of my magic weight-loss formula, but you know it's the key to *yours.*

Most of my genetic results indicate I'm pretty average and not at all a physical dynamo. I'm also likely to experience *more fatigue* while exercising and *slower recovery* than the normal person. I wish I could go back in time and give this report to my gym teachers—it explains a lot.

The lesson from this is that if I gave you a list of the "best" exercises to do, it might be completely wrong for your body. Chances are, you probably already know what types of exercise make *you* feel great, so feel confident that you can answer the question of what exercise is best for you by listening to your body—no DNA test required! My test simply confirmed what I already knew. It's okay to be average, and it's okay for me to sit down when I get tired.

No matter what exercise you decide to do, it's important for all of us to remain active, whether you prefer to be more casual about it like I am or whether you're an elite endurance athlete. Now that we understand how important it is to keep moving, in whatever style feels right to us and may be best for our bodies, let's address specific concerns related to exercise and fasting.

Some of the main questions people ask concern workout timing and fasting. This is such a confusing topic for many, because the conventional advice has been to eat prior to working out (to fuel your workout) and to eat after exercise (to promote muscle growth), and there is even a common misconception out there that if you work out in the fasted state, your body will burn muscle for fuel. Let's get into these topics one by one!

Before I get into the science, though, I want to answer one question: Is there one best time of day to work out? And the answer is this: The best time to work out is the time that fits into your schedule!

I'm sure you've figured this out about me by now: I am all about giving *you* control of how you structure your day and your life. I want *you* to choose the eating window and fasting protocol that feels right to you. I want you to select the foods that make *you* feel great. I want you to do the type of exercise that *you* love. And I want you to work out when *you* feel like working out!

Scientifically, however, there is some compelling evidence that working out in the fasted state is superior to working out in the fed state, despite what you may have been told by the experts up to now. For one thing, autophagy ramps up after exercise,[8] which is one reason why exercising in the fasted state is so beneficial. Even so, if *you* try working out in the fasted state and it makes you feel unwell, or if you find that you're starving all day long and fasting is therefore more difficult, experiment to figure out just the right timing for your body. Also keep in mind that the timing that is right for you now may change as your body becomes more metabolically flexible.

When you consider working out in the fasted state, you may wonder if you will have enough energy. Will you crash and burn?

Remember that fasting ignites our fat-burning superpower, so working out in the fasted state allows us to tap into fat stores for fuel![9] When you can use your stored fat, you have access to an amazing source of steady energy. One caveat—if you are new to IF and haven't yet flipped the metabolic switch, it will be difficult to work out in the fasted state. Give your body time to adjust, and while you wait, stick to easier forms of exercise, such as walking, yoga, and so on. This isn't the time for a HIIT session. Over time, however, you'll train your body to burn fat while exercising in the fasted state. Also, keep in mind that if you are an endurance athlete and therefore at a different level of activity than the average person who is simply trying to get through a Zumba class, you may need different strategies for fueling extended workouts.

Another common question is whether you need to eat right before exercise or right after exercise to prevent your body from breaking down your valuable muscle tissue and using it for fuel. Is that true?

No! Our bodies are not dumb. Think about it! You're working out and using your muscles as you exercise. Is your body going to break down other valuable muscle tissue to fuel your body? Of course not! You have fat stored on your body *for that very purpose*—to fuel your body when needed. It makes no sense that your body would turn to your muscle tissue if fat is readily available, as is the case when we fast clean. When you flip your metabolic switch, your body's shift in fuel sources is a key factor in muscle preservation. When you're fasting, your muscles themselves make the shift from using glucose to using fatty acids during endurance exercise, which leads to increased endurance capacity.[10]

Keep in mind that if you are an endurance athlete who needs to fuel up for something more intense than an average spin class, you may have different needs than I have just discussed. Look for someone who understands both your specific sport and intermittent fasting who can help you train and compete under the ideal conditions for you.

You also may hear that it's necessary to consume protein immediately before or after working out to provide the building blocks your body needs to build new muscle. It sounds plausible, right? Well, is *that* true?

Again, the answer is no. In a 2013 meta-analysis of *all* the research on protein timing and muscle growth, scientists found that there is no need to consume protein immediately before or after a workout and that meal timing made no difference in either muscle growth or muscle strength. The only important factors were having adequate *overall* protein consumption and a sufficient resistance training regimen.[11] So, no need to worry about eating pre- or post-workout! Eat sufficient protein in your daily eating window and you'll be just fine. Don't forget one other important fact—when we fast, our bodies have increased levels of human growth hormone.[12,13] This gives us yet another muscle-building advantage!

Well, what about supplements? These days, everywhere you turn, someone has a fancy supplement to sell you.

Do you need the energy boost of a pre-workout? (You probably can answer this question yourself, thinking back to the answer to previous questions.) During a fasted workout, you will first use stored muscle glycogen to fuel your muscles. Your body also upregulates fat burning. Our bodies have no choice but to turn to stored fat for fuel once we've depleted our glycogen sufficiently! So, no pre-workout needed. (Though I do want to give you some good news. Coffee and/or caffeine appear to have some benefits when used pre-workout; studies show increased speed and endurance and resistance to fatigue.[14] And it's clean-fast approved!)

Do we need a supplement *after* working out to promote muscle building? The answer is no. Just as we don't need to eat immediately before or after working out, we also don't need special supplements surrounding our workout. As I mentioned in chapter 3, research shows us that fasting increases the availability of many compounds within our bodies that are essential for muscle growth, such as carnitine (which increases blood flow to the muscles) and branched-chain amino acids (BCAAs, which prevent muscle breakdown and encourage growth of new muscle tissue).

While you may hear that our bodies can't *make* BCAAs (therefore we have to get them through our foods), our bodies can *recycle* them during the fast, which is why we see an upregulation in their availability during the fast.[15] Despite what you may have heard (probably from someone trying to sell you supplements), our bodies are actually great at recycling amino acids.[16] I found a quote in a scientific journal that really says it all: "There is general agreement that the most important role of autophagy is the supply of amino acids under nutrient-poor conditions."[17] Let me translate this into plain English. When you fast, autophagy takes care of supplying your amino acid needs. So, again! No pre- or post-workout supplements needed! Thanks, autophagy!

I want to give one caveat. If you are a serious bodybuilder, you may have different needs from what I have outlined here. The average person who wants to build muscle through a workout routine is going to be just fine following my advice, but if you are a competitor, look elsewhere for the advice that will help you meet your specific goals.

Now, there is something I need to tell you. Intermittent fasters who are exercising usually find that weight loss is *slower* when they incorporate exercise than when they don't.

WHAT???

Deep breath. No need to panic! Let me explain!

This phenomenon is due to the magic of body recomposition, which I explained in chapter 18. Go back and read that section if you can't remember the specifics.

Body recomposition changes happen for most of us, even those who are *not* doing a formal exercise program. But if you *are* exercising, the effects of body recomposition are even more pronounced. You'll burn fat and build muscle like never before, so don't let the scale get you down. It will be even more important for you to use the other methods for tracking progress, and photos will likely be your most powerful tool.

Before I move on to the next chapter, there is one more thing I want to talk about. Think back to what I told you about fasting in the red flags chapter—you *can* overdo fasting, and if you do, that's not a good thing for your body. Well, the same is true for exercise. You absolutely *can* overdo it. And what's even worse, if you are fasting hard *and* training hard, that may be entirely too much for your body.

I can't tell you what is "too much" for you. However, just as I taught you in previous chapters, you want to make sure you feel great. If, at any time, you start feeling worse and worse, or you develop the urge to binge, those are signs that your body is not happy with what you are doing. Just as I cautioned you to scale back your fasting if you see warning signs, the same is true for exercise. Sometimes, less really is more, whether we are talking about exercise or fasting.

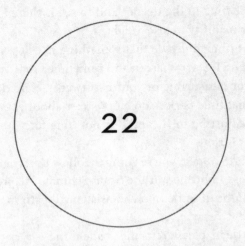

22

WEIGHT LOSS TOO SLOW OR YOU'RE AT A PLATEAU? HOW TO ADJUST AND ADAPT

"Help, Gin! IF isn't working for me!"

First, it's important to consider one thing—intermittent fasting might not be "working" for *weight loss* for you right now, but that doesn't mean it isn't working for health benefits. Revisit chapters 2 and 3 and remember that IF is the health plan with a side effect of weight loss. Of course, most of us came for the weight loss (even though we stick around for the health benefits), so I understand why you would be frustrated if you aren't seeing the weight loss you hope for.

This chapter is for all the IFers out there who have been living the intermittent fasting lifestyle for a while and are not yet seeing any measurable progress, or for those of you who may be at a weight-loss plateau. It's full of strategies that are tried-and-true. I will also tell you when it is time to dig deeper and to see if there is another root cause of your inability to lose weight.

When is it time to decide that something needs tweaking? Think back to the FAST Start chapter and remember that you should not be weighing or measuring for your first twenty-eight days. If you are still within that time period, do NOT stress about your results. Your body is still adjusting to IF, and it is not time for you to worry that your progress is slow.

After the FAST Start, you're going to follow the strategies for measuring progress I outlined in the Scale-Schmale chapter. Give yourself a few months to settle into a consistent IF pattern, and continue to tweak it till it's easy.

As you settle in, please remember one thing—intermittent fasting is not like other things you've done. With "diets" of the past, we usually had spectacular and quick results at the very beginning that then fizzled out, and then we usually started to slowly gain the weight back. With IF, we usually do *not* have that dramatic and quick early loss (though some people do have a *whoosh* of a few pounds during the first couple of weeks).

When we are fasting, our bodies are doing something different; they are learning how to tap into our stored fat. So, the results are pretty much the opposite. We do *not* have those spectacular and quick results. In fact, we frequently see our results begin to pick up slowly, and weight loss may increase as time goes on. (It's true! I lost weight more quickly the closer I got to my initial goal weight of 135 pounds. As I've already told you, at that point, I was eating within a fairly tight eating window, and I had also cleaned up what I was eating, temporarily delaying ultra-processed foods and alcohol, but I was losing weight at an astronomical pace of about *two* pounds per week. Why was the rate of loss so quick? I think the reason was twofold; it was because, first, my body was fully adjusted to intermittent fasting, and I had unleashed my fat-burning superpower, and second, because I was also eating mostly whole foods that worked well for my body.)

Before discussing strategies for increasing weight loss or busting a plateau, I want to mention that there are several groups of people who tend to have very slow initial results when beginning an intermittent fasting protocol.

- **If you have a recent history of dieting, particularly if you were following a restrictive plan: a low-calorie diet, a meal-replacement program (e.g., diet shakes or bars), prescription diet pills, certain "medical weight loss" programs, and so on.**

    If this sounds like you, then you are going to need more time for your body to recover. Think back to the introduction where I discussed the way our bodies adapt to a restrictive diet by slowing metabolic rate. Intermittent fasting is one of your best bets for healing your slow metabolic rate, and an up-and-down-day protocol will likely be a great choice for your body. Go back to that chapter and read the many ways that the up-and-down-day protocol might be structured.

- **If you have been overweight or obese for a long time, if you suffer from PCOS (polycystic ovary syndrome), if you are prediabetic, or if you have type 2 diabetes.**

    If this describes you, then it is likely that your body is severely insulin resistant (and if you have been diagnosed as prediabetic or with type 2 diabetes, then this is definitely going to be true for you). The key is going to be getting your insulin down over time so your body can heal. While fasting is wonderful for lowering insulin levels, you may also need a more structured dietary approach to lower insulin even more. Remember that we need to have lower levels of circulating insulin to tap into our fat stores for fuel during the fast. This is where a low-carb or keto plan can make a positive difference. You may not have to follow a lower-carb plan forever; a combination of low-carb eating and intermittent fasting can reverse your insulin resistance over time, and you may find that you can tolerate more carbs as time goes on and your body heals.

- **If you have recently been gaining weight rapidly.**

    If you have been gaining a lot of weight recently, then that is a sign that something is going on in your body. If this is true for you, when you start IF, you may find that the weight *gain* stops, but you don't *lose* any weight. Think about this for a minute. If you *were* gaining a lot of weight, and now you are *not,* that is a positive step in the right direction. Give your body at *least* three to six months (or even longer!) before you expect any weight loss. At that time, you can start to experiment with some of the tweaks in this chapter.

- **If you take medications linked to weight gain.**

    If you take any medications regularly, go ask Uncle Google for a list of side effects; see if weight gain is a typical side effect for your prescriptions. If so, it can be very difficult to lose weight as long as you take them. Have a conversation with your doctor and/or pharmacist to see if there are any options that may work better for you.

- **If you are hypothyroid.**

    If your thyroid isn't functioning properly, it can be very difficult to lose weight. And here's what's even more frustrating—you can have a thyroid that isn't working up to steam and still have "normal" blood work. This is a very complex issue, and it is unfortunately beyond the scope of this book. I recommend that you find a forward-thinking doctor skilled in all things thyroid to help you figure out exactly what your unique body needs to optimize your thyroid function.

If one of those scenarios sounds like you, then really focus on what I said about your specific situation. If not, keep reading.

If you are beyond the FAST Start phase and at least eight weeks into your intermittent fasting lifestyle, you first need to make sure you are really not making progress before tweaking. Go back to chapter 18, consider all the ways to track your progress, and really examine your data—compare your weekly averages, look at your overall weight trends, see if your measurements are decreasing, try on your honesty pants, and check your comparison photos. If you are making progress—even slow progress—you are successful and don't need to change anything!

If you determine that you are indeed not losing weight (or getting measurably smaller), the good news is that you absolutely can make some tweaks that should make a difference. As I mentioned in a previous chapter, every time you make a change, give it at least two weeks to see what happens. Consider each change to be an experiment along your personal study of one, and don't rush the process. It's best to tweak only ONE thing at a time and to measure your results to see if it is working.

- **First, check your fast. Are you *really* fasting clean?** Go back to the basics—only black and unflavored coffee, plain teas, plain water, and unflavored sparkling waters. Have you been using just a bit of coconut oil or cream in your coffee? Are you drinking flavored waters? Are you adding *anything* to your plain coffee, tea, or water? Are you chewing gum or using breath mints or breath strips? Perhaps it's making more of a difference than you thought. (*YES, IT IS! I promise!*) I can't overemphasize the importance of a clean fast.

  Also, if you *have been* doing IF for a while without fasting clean, once you shift to the clean fast, you may have a period of weight *gain* while your body adjusts to the clean fast. Consider the day you shift to the clean fast as your day 1, and consider the time prior to that as a low-calorie diet, and understand that you weren't actually receiving the metabolic and hormonal benefits of fasting. You'll need some time, and patience is required.

- **Next, be honest with yourself when it comes to food volume.** Remember, even though there are many flaws related to the concept of counting calories to control how much you eat (because your body doesn't work like a laboratory calorimeter), it absolutely is possible to eat so much food that you don't lose weight. If you overeat, your body stores away whatever it can't use now for later.

While intermittent fasting has been shown to increase metabolic rate, it isn't likely to increase it so much that you can overeat day after day. Your goal is to eat until pleasantly satisfied and then stop. If you hope to lose fat, then volume of food does matter. Revisit the appetite correction chapter for strategies that might help you.

• **Examine your food quality.** While I have taught you to *delay* rather than *deny,* that doesn't mean that all foods are working well for your body for weight loss. Think back to chapter 17. Are you eating a diet that is mostly composed of ultra-processed foods? If so, this is an easy thing to tweak. For now, *delay* most of the ultra-processed foods that are in your diet and see what happens. I predict that you'll find amazing appetite correction immediately and also notice that weight loss ramps up quickly.

• **Consider switching up (or tightening up) your fasting regimen.** There are many ways to live an intermittent fasting lifestyle. After much experimentation, I prefer a daily-eating-window approach, but that doesn't mean it's the best approach for you. You may need to try some different strategies to get the scale moving.

If you use the daily-eating-window approach but weight loss is slow, consider tightening it up. I couldn't lose weight with anything longer than a five-hour window, and even a five-hour window is too long for some people. Shorten your eating window for a while, and see if that helps. One suggestion is to use a one- to two-hour window on weekdays and give yourself a longer window (five to eight hours hours) on weekends. As I have said before, it can be helpful to mix things up rather than get into a consistent daily routine that encourages your body to adapt. You can also add one longer fast per week, if you are really motivated. I have seen many people who add one 36-hour or 42-hour full fast once per week and finally start to see results on the scale. Remember to have an up day after a longer fast like this.

Another idea is to incorporate the up-and-down-day approach.

If you have a long dieting history, the up-and-down-day approach may be your best bet for increasing metabolic rate over time. Remember that the key is to have true up days following every down day. You want your body to get the message that you are *not* in any danger of starving.

- **Experiment with different eating styles.** As I taught you in the bio-individuality chapter, we are all different when it comes to what foods work well for our bodies. You may have a body that does better with a lower-carb approach, or perhaps your body will do better with less dietary fat. Experiment! Try a time where you eat fewer carbs, alternated with no carb restriction at all. Or give yourself a few weeks where you eat less fat, alternated with no fat restriction. Really pay attention to how you feel, and see if either intervention makes a difference in your rate of progress.

  Unlike the low-carb or low-fat diets of past decades, I don't want you to rely on ultra-processed carb or fat *replacements.* Instead, focus on real foods that are either lower in carbs or fat. Fake foods are not the answer here; real foods are.

  Also, remember that you don't need to give up foods you love forever. You may be *delaying* excess carbs or excess fat in your diet for a time so that you can lose the excess fat on your body. Once you lose the weight you are hoping to lose, you can experiment with adding foods back in. There is a lot more flexibility in maintenance!

- **Change the time of day of your window.** While most IFers tend to gravitate to an evening eating window, that doesn't mean it's the universally best time to eat. Experiment with other times of day! If you have been having an evening eating window, shift it first to midday and see how that works for you. If you have tried that for a while and it doesn't seem to suit you, shift your window to morning and see what happens. I know several IFers who absolutely thrive with an early-in-the-day eating window! This may prove to be true for you.

If you realize that an earlier eating window doesn't feel right for you, that's fine, too. Try a different tweak from the list.

• **Delay desserts, alcohol, and/or caloric beverages.** This is a big one for me and appears to make all the difference for my body. Remember that when I was initially losing weight in the spring of 2015, I temporarily delayed both desserts and alcohol to get to my goal weight more quickly (I also delayed ultra-processed foods, as I mentioned). I did allow myself to have fresh berries with heavy cream whenever I wanted something sweet, but I didn't add any sweeteners or eat sugary desserts.

I also found that alcohol stalled my weight loss completely. There are two reasons that this is true for me; first, our bodies use the energy from alcohol *first*.[1] If you drink alcohol, then that means that your body will use the energy from the alcohol and then store away any excess energy from the foods you eat (putting the extra carbs into glycogen storage or fat storage and socking the extra fat away into your fat cells).[2] The second issue has to do with appetite. I have also realized that when I drink alcohol, I tend to eat more food (and alcohol's impact on overeating has also been demonstrated in scientific studies). In a 2010 study, they found "significantly more energy was consumed following alcohol than no-alcohol."[3] So, if you are trying to lose weight, alcohol may not be your friend.

Also look at other beverages you may be including during your eating window. Are you choosing caloric beverages (such as sugar-sweetened sodas or sugary lattes)? While you know that I don't want you to count calories (and I have fully explained why), these types of beverages are called "empty calories" for a reason. Delay them for now, and see if that makes a difference.

So now the big question is this: **Which of the strategies from this chapter should you try first?**

Read over them carefully. See if any of them resonate with you and start there. Just as we have an intermittent fasting toolbox, consider these tweaks to be additional tools that you have to choose from. Mix it up!

In a survey within our online support community, intermittent fasters reported that this is how they busted through a plateau of a month or more (in order of number of responses):

- Time and patience

- Altering window length

- Changing time of window

- Lowering carbs

- ADF (alternate-daily fasting, or the up-and-down-day protocol)

- Delaying alcohol

- A weekly 36- to 48-hour fast

- 23:1

- Delaying sugar

- Delaying processed foods

- Adding exercise

- 5:2 (five up days, two down days per week)

- 4:3 (four up days, three down days per week)

These strategies are all tried-and-true, and with time and patience, most people are usually able to see the weight loss they are hoping for. But: **What happens if you are doing everything right, you've tried the tweaks from this chapter, and you are *still* not seeing any measurable progress after several months to a year?**

Some people, particularly in the groups I mentioned at the beginning of this chapter, may have bodies that are more resistant to weight loss. You may need one thing more than any other: **TIME.**

Yes, you need to give it time.

It may feel like your body is broken and beyond repair.

But remember this—your body didn't put on the excess weight overnight, and the hormonal changes that need to occur behind the scenes also aren't going to happen overnight. Keep on fasting consistently, keep fasting clean, and eat quality foods. Let your body heal. Pay attention to how various foods make you feel, and select foods that make you feel good. Focus on the other positive benefits you can detect, and trust the process.

There are people who live an intermittent fasting lifestyle for *months* before seeing scale movement. Trust that once your body is ready, you should begin to see progress.

Never forget that over time, even slow progress adds up. A pound here, a pound there—eventually, you should lose the excess fat at the speed that is right for *your* body.

Also, please understand that a plateau doesn't mean that you are doomed to never lose another pound or that you are about to yo-yo up again. Instead, think of a plateau as a way for your body to establish a new set point before it's ready to lose more fat.

I have a few final thoughts that I want to leave you with. In our intermittent fasting communities, we always say "trust the process." But when is it time to dig deeper beyond IF alone?

If you have been trying to lose weight with IF for a year or more, and you have tried the tweaks from this chapter and are still not seeing results, it's time to look more closely at what could be preventing your body from accessing your stored fat for fuel. (I'm not talking to you, turtles! If you are losing weight slowly, you *are* successful.)

To anyone who is struggling with the weight-loss side of the equation: IF will help you with weight loss *only* if it addresses the reason(s) *you* are overweight.

Think about that again: **IF works for weight loss only if it addresses the reason(s)** *your* **body is holding on to the weight.**

When IF does not address your specific issue(s), that's when you need to dig deeper to figure out what is keeping your body from releasing the weight.

- An undiagnosed thyroid issue?

- Food sensitivities?

- Underlying health conditions?

- Going through menopause?

- Stress?

- Lack of sleep, or shift work?

- Medications that are related to weight gain?

Never forget that obesity is a complicated problem, because our bodies are extremely complex. You solve the problem only when you address *your* issue(s).

Over the years, I've realized that IF really is the health plan with a side effect of weight loss, but that doesn't mean that you won't have to dig in to your own health issues on a deeper level to figure out what is holding you back personally.

This is really important to understand.

So, trust the process in the sense that IF is good for your body and that it's likely helping you achieve better health overall. Yes. But that doesn't mean it is all *you* may have to do to figure out your own complicated body. Remember that weight loss is a billion-dollar industry—$68 *billion* in 2017 alone. If it were simple, no one would be overweight. The truth of the matter is that it's not simple.

If you have tweaked and tweaked and are still struggling to lose weight long term, I would encourage you to find a forward-thinking health care practitioner who is willing to dig deep with you. This is not always easy, as I recall a couple of my own doctors who were only too happy to prescribe diet pills. I was only too happy to *accept* them, in fact, because I didn't know everything I know now. (Boy, do I wish I could travel back in time and hand my younger, struggling self a copy of this book. I would have saved myself a lot of angst.)

The good news is that there are *so many* excellent doctors out there who are willing to do the work alongside you. When you have tried everything, rest assured that something is going on in your body, and it's not your fault.

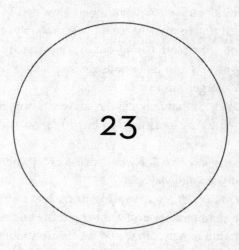

23

MAINTENANCE:
IF FOR L*IF*E

One of the best things about intermittent fasting is that maintenance is like *nothing* you have ever tried before, and most IFers go on to maintain within a healthy weight range long term with little effort or struggle!

The first big question: How do you know when you are there? How do you know that you're actually "in maintenance"? Believe it or not, this can be a difficult question to answer for many people.

When you begin IF, you probably have an idea of what your "goal weight" should be. Actually, I would like you to reconsider that idea, particularly as you begin to get closer and closer to that magic number.

Let me tell you my story here. Initially, when I weighed 210, I wanted to get down to 135 pounds. I chose that number because I remembered feeling really good about my body when I weighed 128, but that seemed like an impossible goal. 135 was 75 pounds down, which seemed like a nice round number. I wanted to fit into a size 6, which seemed *tiny* to my 16W self. I was probably actually 18W, if you want to know the truth (shout-out to you, stretchy clothes, that I was squeezing myself into like a sausage in a casing, refusing to buy anything with a larger number on the tag).

In March of 2015, that magical day arrived: I weighed 135 on the scale! I marched to my local mall to buy my new wardrobe! Size 6, here I am!

Except I was *not* a size 6. I was a size 4 everywhere I went. That was fun! (Vanity sizing? Maybe.)

I bought *so many clothes* that spring, and I felt beautiful. I declared myself to be in maintenance and went about the business of figuring out what my maintenance plan would be. (More about choosing your maintenance plan in a minute!)

In the spring of 2016, after a year of maintaining my weight within my goal range (give or take a few pounds), I decided I no longer desired to have my morning mood depend upon what number the scale showed to me. The last day I weighed, I registered a 132.5 on the scale, and on that day, I put my scale away on a very high shelf and didn't get on it again for fourteen months.

Over that fourteen-month period, I continued to slowly lose fat. In fact, my size 4 clothes began to get looser and looser, and I found that I needed size *2* clothes, and even size *0* clothes. Yep. I went down *two more* jeans sizes over that fourteen-month period!

One day, I was feeling very brave, and I decided to get the scale back down from the top shelf to see how much more weight I had lost. I felt so much slimmer, and my clothes were smaller; surely, I weighed 125 at the very most. I got onto the scale, exhaled, and . . . 130.8. WHAT?!?!?! Where was the 125 (or lower) that I expected to see? I started to think diet-y thoughts. What could I do to get that number down to 125? How could I lose more weight to get to the *new* goal I had come up with in my head: 125?

I was MAD. And I was MAD that I was MAD.

You see, I had lost *two sizes,* and I expected to be rewarded for that feat by seeing a special number on the scale. Forget about the fact that I was standing there in my size 0 jeans. (Okay, I was actually naked, because I was weighing myself . . . and nobody weighs themselves while wearing jeans, but you get my point.)

I threw my very expensive Bluetooth scale into the garbage that very day, and I haven't weighed myself since. (And when I go to the doctor, I ask them not to tell me.)

The point of the story is this:

I was living in my goal *body*, and my actual *weight* was irrelevant. I knew I didn't need to be any smaller than I was at that point. Sure, I still have curves and squishy areas—I believe women are supposed to have squish and curves, by the way—but did I really need to lose 5.8 more pounds to get to 125? Did I *need* to be a size 00? Of course not!

I was smaller and leaner at 130.8 than I had been years previously at 128 pounds. I still own some jeans and dresses from back then, in fact. The jeans that fit me at 128 were *loose* and there was a gap around the waist, even though I weighed almost 3 pounds more. The dresses that fit me at 128 pounds were loose! Yep. My 130.8-pound body was smaller than my 128-pound body had been.

What's the point of this story? It is to reiterate this concept: instead of choosing a goal *weight,* choose a goal *body.* Pick a body size that will make you happy and take the focus off the scale. Like me, you may never get to that mythical number that sounds so good in your head. Like me, you may find you are *leaner* and *smaller* at a higher weight than you were in the past! Thank you, body recomposition! You have lost fat and built muscle, and that makes such a difference in your size! And, like me, you can learn to love your imperfections and accept that most of us will still have some squishy bits, because we are human and not bikini models. (You may actually be a bikini model, in which case, scratch that.)

Once you decide that you are getting close to your goal body, you may wonder if you need to change what you are doing to maintain your weight. Should you lengthen your eating windows? Have fewer down days? Stop intermittent fasting completely?

While it's true that you can be a bit more relaxed in maintenance, you won't want to relax *too* much . . . or too soon! When you first reach your goal, stick to the protocol you've been using to lose weight and focus on listening to your hunger and satiety cues. You may find that you have increased hunger because you're at an ideal weight for your body (thanks, appestat!). If so, honor that increased hunger, and you'll settle in within a maintenance range that works well for you.

If you ever find that you are losing *more* weight than you want to lose, it will be time to lengthen your eating window a bit. Notice I said *a bit*. You'll want to experiment to find just the right window that works for weight stability.

As you live your life in maintenance, you may also worry about weight regain. That is a legitimate concern because we are used to every diet we did in the past that came along with weight regain over time—the dreaded yo-yo effect that most of us have experienced.

Intermittent fasting helps to protect our bodies from the metabolic slowdown that would lead to weight regain. That's a good thing! But that doesn't mean that you are immune to weight regain.

Let me explain.

Once you successfully reach your goals (thanks to intermittent fasting!), you may be tempted to relax your eating window over time. That is absolutely okay as long as you are also able to maintain your new size! Unfortunately, however, you may find that you have relaxed it to the point where you are slowly regaining weight.

The good news is that the intermittent fasting strategies that helped you *lose* the weight will still be there to help you *maintain* it.

This is how it looks for me. I am very flexible now, and I no longer even count hours or track my eating window. But I do keep a close eye on how my clothes fit. Remember the term *honesty pants* from chapter 18? I have a pair that I pull out from time to time. They are size 0 and have absolutely no stretch or give. If I see a little extra muffin top going on, I know that it's time to rein myself in a little bit.

When I am honest with myself, I always know what to tweak. For me, that usually means I'll have less wine and shorter windows for a while until I'm fitting nicely into those pants again. Even though I don't weigh, I am always keeping tabs on my size, and I'm not going to allow myself to outgrow those honesty pants.

Perhaps the scale is a more useful tool than honesty pants for you, but don't let it be the only one you rely on, especially if you are doing any sort of exercise. You may see an increase on the scale that reflects an increase in muscle mass. You should also continue to rely on your own version of honesty pants and take comparison photos from time to time.

If you do see that you're gaining a little fluff, be completely honest with yourself, just as I am. I *always* can put my finger on what is going on. (This is a teacher trick, by the way. If you say to a kid, "What do *you* think you did wrong?" the kid *always* knows the answer to the question and will either tell you or glare at you, which is equally satisfying because you know they are thinking about their own behavior.)

So, if you notice you are gaining a little weight, ask yourself: **What do I think I may be doing differently that could have caused this weight regain?**

Are you eating *more* food now? Have you changed *what* you're eating? Have you started having longer windows on weekends? Are you drinking more alcohol? Having desserts more frequently? These are a few of the common issues that turn into slippery slopes for many of us.

One important caveat—if you know that nothing has changed in your IF approach but you are still gaining weight unexpectedly, it may be time to revisit chapter 22 to see if you may have something else going on. This could range from a new medication linked to weight gain, stress, a round of antibiotics (that affected your gut microbiome balance), thyroid issues, and so on. Consider working with a medical professional who can help you figure out what may be going on. Above all else, never forget that while the body is incredibly complex, unexpected weight gain is a sign that something is going on that needs your attention, and it doesn't mean it is your fault (or that IF has failed you).

Maintenance can be terrifying to those of us with decades of failed diets stretching behind us, but it is also thrilling to discover that year after year, you'll become more confident that your new body is here to stay. As 2015 turned into 2016, then 2017, 2018, 2019, and 2020, I have continued to marvel at how easy maintenance truly is when compared to all the diets I did in the past. Throughout all the years of my IF maintenance, there has not been one moment where I needed to buy bigger clothes because I was gaining weight, even as I go through menopause. By remaining truthful with myself, keeping track of my size (thanks to my honesty pants), and continuing to live an intermittent fasting lifestyle, I am certain that I have finally figured this thing out, once and for all.

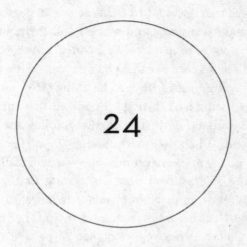

24

SHARE WITHOUT FEAR

Many new intermittent fasters are nervous about sharing intermittent fasting with others. Will people think you are crazy??? Will you get lectures from well-meaning friends and family members? (Actually, maybe! I did. But if that happens, I want to teach you how to handle it with poise and confidence!)

As you can imagine, I *love* to talk to people about intermittent fasting. These days, I have noticed that more and more people have heard about it when I bring it up. Most people have seen a magazine article or a news snippet, or perhaps they have a friend, family member, or acquaintance who has had great success. Now when I mention it, more people have heard of intermittent fasting than have *not* heard of it.

And if that weren't enough, I have two pieces of evidence that will convince you that intermittent fasting is, indeed, mainstream.

First, it's the rise of intermittent fasting products. Remember the low-fat craze of the 1990s? We knew it was big-time when every food product boasted that it was fat-free. The same can be said for the low-carb era (all the Atkins bars and snacks) and the popularity of the keto diet (every coffee shop offers "keto coffee"). Well, the other day, I saw an ad for a new snack bar that you can "eat" while you are doing intermittent fasting. After I stopped laughing (How gullible do they think we are? Eating isn't fasting.), I realized that the rise of these products is a very good sign! You can always follow the money to see what is on trend. When they start making "food" for "fasting," you know there's a large market. (Promise me you won't fall for it. Repeat after me: Eating isn't fasting. Eating isn't fasting. Eating isn't fasting.)

The second exciting piece of evidence is more scientific. In the 2018 Food and Health Survey conducted by the International Food Information Council, they reported that 36 percent of consumers claimed to follow an "eating pattern" of some sort during the prior calendar year.[1] Of those following an eating pattern, guess what the *top* self-reported eating pattern was? If you guessed "intermittent fasting," you are a winner! (You're still a winner even if you didn't guess that, because you are here reading a book about intermittent fasting, and if that doesn't make you a winner, I don't know what does.)

If you take the time to look on page 26 of that report, there is a graphic showing all the most-reported eating patterns. Intermittent fasting is right there at the top. A full *10 percent* of the participants following a structured eating plan in 2018 reported that they were doing intermittent fasting, more than any other diet or eating pattern. It ranked higher than Paleo. Higher than gluten-free. Higher than vegetarian or vegan. Higher than keto. Whoa! Mainstream, baby.

So! Now you know—intermittent fasting is no longer in the shadows. It's so mainstream that it was the number one self-reported "eating pattern" of 2018, and the marketers are ready to sell you fasting bars for your fast.

And remember that if people have questions, you don't need to have all the answers, and you certainly do *not* have to spend your time defending what you do. Nope. If you find that someone is still giving you a hard time about intermittent fasting, or if they say it isn't "healthy," lend them your copy of *Fast. Feast. Repeat.* and tell them you'll be happy to discuss it with them once they have read the book. (Or better yet, buy them their own copy. They probably won't return yours to you anyway, so go ahead and save the step.)

I'm happy to explain fasting to them on your behalf through my book. And if they aren't willing to learn, you can release their thoughts from your mind. *You* know what you are doing. *You* know intermittent fasting is the health plan with a side effect of weight loss, and *you* are confidently living the intermittent fasting lifestyle.

If you tell someone that you are an intermittent faster and they reply with criticisms such as, "Of course you're losing weight! You're on the starvation diet!" or the famous "Well, if I stopped eating, I would lose weight, too," one strategy is to confuse them with science-y words:

"Well, Bob, I have been interested in ways I could increase autophagy in my body ever since the 2016 Nobel Prize in Medicine was awarded for research on the health and longevity benefits of upregulating autophagic processes in the body. I'm sure that you know that intermittent fasting is the best way to do that, which is why I do it."

Crickets.

No one can argue with science-y words that contain phrases like *Nobel Prize in Medicine* and *upregulating autophagic processes.* I promise.

So, lead with the health benefits. After all, we all know that intermittent fasting is the health plan with a side effect of weight loss.

And eventually, when they see your stunning success firsthand, *they* will be coming to *you* for your secrets. That is the way it worked for me. People who had watched me struggle for *years* as I tried crazy diet after crazy diet were waiting for me to crash and burn with IF, as well. When year after year went by, and I maintained a loss of over eighty pounds, suddenly Gin wasn't so crazy anymore.

Overall, I would say that having confidence in what you are doing may be the number one most important predictor of success. When you understand that intermittent fasting is linked to health and longevity, you know that what you are doing is good for your body. And when you know that what you are doing is good for your body, you aren't ashamed or embarrassed to tell others about it, and you also don't feel like you need to hide what you are doing.

We are on the cusp of a revolution! We have the opportunity to change the world together! When we #ShareWithoutFear, we may plant the seed that grows into vibrant health for our friends and loved ones. There is no better feeling than that.

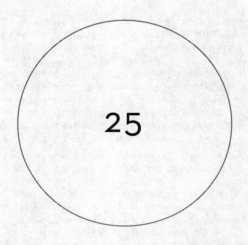

25

"WHAT I WISH I KNEW"

Intermittent fasting is a lifestyle that will change your life in more ways than you can imagine. In this chapter, IFers from around the world share their words of wisdom. Come back to this chapter whenever you need a pep talk or inspiration!

Nancy Miller	This is a do-able Way of Life! You can start TODAY because there are no special foods, equipment, or memberships to purchase. If you can open your eyes in the morning and fix yourself a cup of unflavored black coffee or tea, or a glass of water, you'll be on your way!
Krista from Hingham, MA	Hunger pains are often more mental (including boredom) than physical. Find something else to do and then see if you still feel hungry after. In my case, I believe I feel most hungry just before my body goes into fat-burning mode. While I can't measure this scientifically, the pattern is so consistent that I now welcome that "hunger" and see it as a positive sign . . . and it goes away pretty quickly. This, and I can't believe I like drinking hot water!

cont.

Heidi in NY	What I wish I knew before starting IF is to pace myself. So many of us start IF after years (decades?) of dieting, and that diet mentality is hard to let go. In a diet, one is used to either seeing or not seeing obvious results (on the scale) within a few days or a week. Understanding that IF is a years-long process—even a lifelong learning process—has helped me tremendously. I've also learned how important health goals are in addition to the scale or size measurements. The perspective that comes with that understanding has helped me to be so much more patient and forgiving with myself than I've been before. It also has helped me feel much more accomplished with small goals, which add up.
NJ IFer	I've been fighting my weight since age 8. I'm a physician, and was taught that it was important to eat 5 times a day to prevent slowing of metabolism. The opposite is true for me as a post-menopausal woman. I wish I knew about IF earlier, as, honestly, I had lost all hope. I fought hunger all the time. Now with IF, I've had appetite correction, I'm effortlessly maintaining a 64 lb. weight loss, I'm mid-range BMI and my mind is even sharper. I love this way of life. I also wish I knew that it would take me 2-3 months to adapt. Everyone said 2 weeks but it was definitely months, but now . . . it's so easy. It's worth the process!
Crystal from Tennessee	Starting out I wish I had known how much coffee really helps! I have never been a coffee drinker and I decided to try it just to see why everyone suggested it. It took me four days of having one cup a day to finally start to like it! Those first four days were horrible!!! I gagged the whole time! Now I drink around 4 cups a day and I love it!
Lisa Breeden	Something I wish I knew when just starting IF is how easy it was. When I first heard about IF, I thought cool—I can barely keep it together through 3 meals and 2 snacks so I would never be able to do IF, let alone one meal a day. I started very gentle with an 8-hour window, with no expectations of going any further. After about 2 weeks I went to a 6-hour window just because I was currently going to the gym and wanted to eat and give my food time to digest before working out. Before long, my hunger was adjusting and I naturally went down to a 3- or 4-hour window, which is where I am now. I have not pushed myself through this process. It has been a gradual thing that I have let my body lead me through. I have been surprised with the appetite correction and how good I feel with this lifestyle.
Becca W	IF is a wonderful gift to give yourself. By living an IF lifestyle you're giving your body a chance to heal and to rest. Your body spends a lot of time digesting food and by fasting you're giving your body a chance to take care of healing other parts of your body.
Laura G.	I wish I knew that there are different kinds of "hunger." The kind that comes from habit or emotions can and should be ignored. When you start to feel hungry, ask yourself if this is actual hunger or is it coming from an external place. Are you bored? Sad? Anxious? Then the hunger is most likely emotional . . . ignore it. Does it grow and grow and not go away? Then it's time to refuel your body.

Gail Rains	I wish I had known how amazingly simple it is to live the intermittent fasting lifestyle! No food restrictions, no membership fees, no food-prepping, no weighing, no products to purchase! Simply fast, feast, repeat.
Amy from Oklahoma	I wish I had read about the clean fast before I started my IF journey. I was just winging it from hearing successful stories from friends. I have seen much better results with following a clean fast and sticking to my window. I also wish I had started sooner. I was so worried that it would be too hard and I would be HANGRY all the time but it was so easy for me and I embraced the hunger and learned to listen better to my body. I LOVE how easy this is for me. I am a mom of 4 and not having to come up with a healthy meal for breakfast has been life changing! Just try it, you won't regret it!
Laura Baukol	I wish I knew about how important the clean fast is! I started IF but was still having cream in my coffee and peppermint or citrus in my water. I learned about the importance of a clean fast a few weeks after starting IF. The graphic is so helpful! I switched to fasting clean, and it made IF easier and more productive for me. I'm not spiking my insulin during my fast, and I'm allowing my body to burn through my glycogen stores to access my fat stores for energy. I have such energy during the day now! I feel great with IF, and I'm glad I switched to a clean fast! I now consider my IF start date the day I started fasting clean. Thank you, Gin!
Karen Thomas	Don't give up!! It takes a while for your body to get it. Go slow and remember it's not a diet, it's a lifestyle
Madeline Colón from Cleveland, OH	I started this journey almost 11 months ago. I wished I knew, as a binge eater/food addict, what and how to eat, and what signs to listen to from our bodies to see if we're doing it right or wrong. I started by doing IF 14/10 to see how my body reacted and for the first couple of days my stomach was doing all kinds of noises. I calmed those noises with water. After two months I was a pro. Then I decided to increase my fasting time by two hours and my body adapted well because I was consistent and patient. You need to enjoy the process. I healed my body and soul with intermittent fasting. I'm no longer a binge eater/food addict!
Kristie from Clarkston, MI	I wish I knew sooner that making such a simple change in my life like IF could have such a profound impact on my weight, my state of mind, my health, my energy, and my overall well-being.
Lori in North Texas	I wish I had known that it is ok to trust my body. I didn't gain all my weight overnight and I wasn't going to lose it overnight either. I wish I had known how much I would love the freedom IF has given me. I wish I had known that the scales don't really tell the whole truth. My body does. I wish I had known about IF 30 years ago!
Gina from Portland, Oregon	Have a plan but be flexible! Start out with whatever window you feel you can successfully accomplish and stick to that until you're ready to increase your time. BUT it's also key to remember that this is not a diet! If you open your window early or close it late a day or two, it's not a crisis. Build those fasting muscles and be kind to yourself as you begin to listen to your body.

cont.

Isha Sharma	Take pictures every week at least. The way the clothes fit changes much more quickly than the number on the scale. It is very encouraging to see your back fat disappearing! Also, keep trying on your 'smaller outfits.' I was very surprised to fit in jeans 2 sizes smaller in only about 6 weeks!
Brooke Steckert	Be flexible. Listen to your body and intuition. IF works, but it's not magical with strict rules. Your body knows what you need and when you need it so try different things and you'll KNOW when you have found what works best for you.
FredRNTT	I wish I knew the power and impact of non-scale victories. How my desire to lose weight would turn into my being healthier and feeling better at age 58 than I ever had previously. Nor could I have imagined that I would become an inspiration to so many others who are also IFing.
Kyla Deatherage	I wish I knew how easy it was to take control of the one aspect of my life that has been out of control since childhood. With IF I have found sanity with food, and strength to tackle it one day, one fast at a time. I just wish I knew about IF years before I did, before the physical and mental damage of a lifetime of being overweight had set in.
Stacy Owen	When I first started I was still in a "diet" mentality. I had quick, and pleasantly surprising results in the first week. The second week was not as successful. So, I naturally became frustrated and figured this plan was just like all other fad diets, and for a brief second reconsidered continuing. THEN I did what I was stubborn about giving up . . . no more creamer and flavored water during my fasting period. Wow, what a huge difference that made! A clean fast makes more difference than I had realized and it wasn't that hard to adjust. I would have creamer in my window but then eventually didn't even want it anymore. I drink plain mineral water because the carbonation helps with tummy grumbles and will have a flavored water in my window if I feel like it. This has been the easiest thing I've ever done to lose weight, but I feel so much better too and that is a super bonus in my book!
Susanna Patten	When I began intermittent fasting, I wish I had truly believed the notion and truth that I would live this lifestyle for the rest of my life. I knew I would see improvements in my health over months, but I didn't necessarily think I would maintain my new style of eating and living life years later. The benefits keep showing up. One month I will see my weight drop, another I might maintain but my skin is tighter and I can tell my muscle tone has improved. Intermittent fasting gives consistently like no other way of living!
Stephanie Conley	I wish I knew that it was okay to give myself permission to listen to my body. That I don't need to eat just because it's "time to eat." My body knows when it's hungry (in reference to years of forcing myself to eat breakfast because I was taught I needed to.)
Raksha	I wish I knew about this way of life a long time ago. The word "fasting" throws some people off. It is not starving yourself. It is delaying food while your body processes existing sugars and fats. I like the versatility

of the program. There is no 'messing up.' You just move on and start and close your window again. And I like the idea of being able to work up to the fasting schedule to fit your needs, abilities and personal schedule. Even my doctor is on board with this program. Nothing out there comes close to this type of program. I am thrilled to be on this journey and look forward to losing inches, maintaining a healthy weight and regulating things like sugars, cholesterol, blood pressure etc. that need vigilance in the advancing age. Thank you for this AHA! moment!!!!!

Andrea from Warwickshire, UK	We are told to eat frequently and promised cures with every new diet and health fad which come along. But the human body knows exactly what to do and has plenty of resources to fuel itself without always needing food. Listen to the hunger signals, are they actually because of habit or boredom? Consider what your body needs in terms of good healthy food but don't deny yourself anything as long as it's in moderation and in your window. Listen to the satiety signals, are you feeling full? Stop and allow your body to digest and heal with the next fast. This is a lifestyle which frees you from everything you have been told before. You will benefit from so much more than weight loss, including body recomposition and much more energy.
Michelina from Australia	I wish I had known that it's ok to be hungry. That we don't always need to be feeding that hunger. I think back and realize that I was rarely ever hungry for long because I was snacking throughout the day. When was my body ever given a chance to use its stored fuel? I kept topping up the reserves without giving it a chance to use the stored fuel it had. IF just seems to be a more efficient way of using your body to its best advantage.
Kim from Colorado	This new way of life is truly life changing. I started IF on the advice of my doctor to kick start my metabolism after gaining weight during menopause, but the true benefit has been my increase in energy, and decrease in joint pain and headaches. I am 51 years old, down 22 lbs. since starting in August, and I haven't felt/looked this good in 20 years. Thank you, Gin!
Betsy Maness	That it isn't just about weight loss, it can help improve chronic conditions. I have severe rheumatoid arthritis and have seen a good improvement in my pain levels. IF is for everyone!
Ellen from Chicagoland	I wish I knew that I needed to judge my journey on its own merits and not to compare myself with others. I wish I had the confidence to bust out the tape measure and track that way, because the scale doesn't always move and it can be discouraging. I wish I knew how to talk about IF confidently with others so I wouldn't feel I had to defend my new way of eating. And I wish I knew that more than what I eat, it's the support that I find in groups and through friends that make the journey possible. I'm losing weight, slowly, and I'm eating all the things. And if it takes me 3 years to lose the entirety of what I'd like to lose, so be it. I'd rather live sanely than try to crash diet into a number on a scale that my body and brain cannot maintain. #IFforlife

cont.

Nana to four	I wish I knew that it's a lifestyle I could do so easily. Having my window close when I do (8:00 PM) stops me from snacking at night which was always my downfall. Also I can be flexible depending on my life at the time—I have not ever had a day when I haven't fasted!
Leslie from Portland	I wish I'd known that Intermittent Fasting would be a slow process and that the 'delay' might mean I have to delay not just for a few hours, but for a few months with certain foods until I've reached my goal weight.
Katie Graham	This is the ONLY thing I have tried for weight loss that has worked long term and has ultimately changed my relationship with food. I am in control of the food not the other way around. I challenge anyone who wants to lose weight to just at least give it a try.
DC Craig	Fasting clean is the key. It becomes very easy once you've practiced it for a while! Fasting dirty just isn't worth it because you feel a lot of hunger. (At least I did.) Also, be your own friend. You wouldn't judge your friend harshly for choices made or body shape, so treat yourself the same way as you would a friend. Be supportive and kind to yourself and you'll find your whole mind-set shift toward the positive. Be happy and rejoice that you are taking steps to become the best version of yourself!
Natalie Kelly	I wish I had known that intermittent fasting would be the most powerful thing I've ever done. I certainly didn't expect that IF would affect every aspect of my life and that the longer I did it, the easier it would become and the more amazing the results would be. It has not only enabled me to lose weight, but it also helped me achieve a higher level of physical, mental, emotional, and spiritual well-being than I've ever experienced before. It's the best thing I've ever done.
Tamara Powell	Please be patient. You won't see results immediately and that can be discouraging. Give it time to work the process and allow your body to adjust. Keep the fast clean. If you have a bad day, don't beat yourself up over it. Just take it one day at a time, hour by hour. Be proud of yourself!
Faster from a New York beach town	I thought I couldn't live without food. I thought I would get shaky or weak or mentally distressed if I "needed" food and didn't or couldn't eat. So I always had a nut bar or other snack in the car or in my bag, and never went more than a few hours without eating or snacking on something. I used to be very trim and over the years, extra pounds, which I hate, had crept up and stayed on me. One day I read about IF and on a whim I just waited 16 hours before eating again . . . And then again the next day, and the next. What I did not realize was this: Thinking about food all the time made me enjoy my food LESS. Great foods like crisp pickles and excellent veggies—"low calorie" and "allowed" in my psyche—were not that desirable, because things like chocolate and sweets were restricted, and therefore, "treats" to be desired. Now that I have been fasting for about 4 months, my appetite is gradually correcting itself. To my relief and happiness, I WANT GOOD FOOD. That's what I WANT to eat. I'm not tempted in the same way anymore.

	I had not known it, but thinking about food all the time—evaluating what to eat and when to eat and can I eat that thing—was tyranny. What a blessed relief to be rid of it. For anyone who is starting out—just start! Do it. Before you know it, you will be over the hump, and wonder how you ever ate the way you did before. This will become and feel natural and good. You will be surprised how—even though you thought eating gives you energy—it actually makes you sluggish. You will feel great and fasting will become easy: the way you want to be.
Amy Klitsner	I wish I knew that doing IF would help reduce inflammation and hence help reduce my chronic spine pain significantly. I have been in pain for over 20 years since a terrible car accident in 1994 in which I ruptured the discs in my lower spine. I have been on painkillers for most of those years to control my chronic spine pain after 4 failed spine surgeries. Since doing IF I have been able to get off almost all of my painkillers and am in significantly less pain. It's miraculous.
Missi Geswein	I wish I knew that IF wasn't nearly as scary as it sounds. I love food, so for me, it was overwhelming to think about not eating for so many hours a day—it sounded TERRIBLE. And to lose my beloved creamer and Stevia . . . that made it pretty difficult. After the first few days, though, it was a piece of cake (with ice cream—I can do that in my window)! I've been on this fasting high for 60+ days now (still a newbie) but I truly do not see myself going back on this way of life. I've lost weight, inches, and that diet mentality is slowly starting to fade. <3
Heather P from Fayetteville	1. You're about to embark on a journey that will change your life in a myriad of ways. Please start slowly and build your fasting muscle which will build your health to levels you never thought possible. 2. When things seem like they're not working, that's when the real work is taking place at the cellular level so trust the process! 3. Fast clean EVERY DAY no matter how long or short your fasting period. 4. Say GOODBYE to DIET MENTALITY and jump for joy, shout to the mountaintops, etc. that you NEVER have to do another fad diet . . . EVER!
Jenna Higham	By trusting the process and practicing patience, you will begin to see that Intermittent Fasting resets your life in all areas. All the damage and distress caused by years of constantly eating mixed with constantly dieting slowly but surely disappears and a major sense of calm and clarity appears. But remember this—pharmaceutical and diet industries are worth billions of dollars and everyone just keeps getting sicker and sicker. This lifestyle costs absolutely NOTHING and can even save you money! [Insert Dr. Evil laugh] We've won!
Kathy Hunter	When I started my IF journey I wish that I could have known how profoundly and deeply this was going to heal so many different areas in my life. I have learned that this way of life is not about food, but rather how I see and relate to myself, how I cope with stress and how I show up for

cont.

	myself. The weight has become secondary because for the first time in years I feel comfortable in my own skin and like I have found my way back home to where I belong. It's fun to watch my body get smaller, my skin to get clearer, my eyes to get brighter, but the pot of gold for me is that I now have a loving, honest and transparent relationship with myself and with food. The calm that has bestowed me with this way of life is something that I previously didn't know was within my reach. I'm so very grateful for Gin and the online community for guiding me home.
Megan from California	I had so many non-scale victories (NSVs) from intermittent fasting in the 5 months before I saw any weight loss! I started sleeping better, dry skin issues on my face resolved, I was able to take my wedding ring off for the first time in years, no more plantar fasciitis in the mornings, I lost inches around the waist (and saw other signs of body recomposition), experienced calmer digestion, felt freedom from guilt around food (!), and my body told me it was ready to start exercising for the first time in years. All BEFORE I lost any weight! There are so many healing benefits of intermittent fasting. Focusing on the scale only can be detrimental in the beginning because it can distract you from all the other benefits you might start noticing in your body.
Teresa from Ecuador	After easing into fasting with a few days of 12:12, then over 2 weeks of 14:10 (lost 10 pounds), I was transitioning to 16:8 today. At 16 hours, I wasn't hungry. So I waited . . . At 19.5 hours my body said, "hey it's time to eat!" And what did I want? Not ice cream or bread, but tunafish! I never before even liked tunafish! I didn't really believe that my hunger and cravings would dissipate, and that my body would tell me what healthier foods I really need. This is awesome!
Lauren Wolcott	I wish I'd known there are some side effects but also that they pass. I frequently search the online support group because every question has already been asked by that group. I had headaches the first week & I get flushed at a certain hour mark . . . bodies are weird & the variety of ways they react is astounding. So I guess I would have liked to know: if you experience something weird, don't panic.
Andrea Oliveau	If you are a "dieter" and coming to IF, there is this adjustment period where you want to eat all the things you have denied yourself for years. Eat them! I came from a paleo and gluten-free background, and while I still stay gluten-free, adding grains back into my life has been amazing. Pasta, pizza, toast, are all things I felt guilty about before. Now with IF, I eat them and enjoy them, guilt-free. While your body is going through this adjustment period, you may gain weight. That's totally OK, it will eventually come off. A few weeks after adding these foods back in, you will realize that you can have them whenever you want, and the novelty will wear off. You will gravitate toward healthier choices. There is also a learning curve to figuring out what your body needs, in terms of the amount of food you eat. For a while, I was eating two full meals a day (in a four- to five-hour eating window) and I couldn't figure out why I wasn't losing

	weight. I finally realized I probably only needed a snack at that first meal! I'm a bit embarrassed how long it took me to figure that out. ;) Now I eat a snack to open my window and a nice meal, and I'm losing at a steady rate. You are on a journey of discovering YOU. Enjoy!
Elaine Thomas	IF is not a quick fix diet. It takes time to have results. Stay away from the scale and do measurements instead. Always take before pictures to compare. Don't compare yourself to others' weight loss. We are all different.
Cristy from Marietta	First, I wish I had known about this way of life years ago! I wish I'd known that it is possible to have a healthy relationship with food and still feel great, and lose weight in the process.
Becky from Tucson	I am a runner. I love moving my body in the great outdoors! I love training for things I find challenging and proving I'm stronger than I thought. Before starting IF, I was always curious and a little worried about if I'd be able to run in the mornings if my eating window was in the evenings. I wish I had known that YES, as long as you let your body slowly get used to the fasting routine, it is positively LOVELY to go for a run or walk in the morning and fast clean until dinner. I attribute a lot of success from my last marathon to IF. Having trained my body to excel at burning fat for fuel, I didn't "hit the wall" that many runners encounter at mile 20. Anyone who likes to run, walk, and/or hike—IF can make you enjoy yourself even more!
Leah H. from Des Moines	I wish I had known about Intermittent Fasting years ago. It almost feels as if I wasted so much of my life being constantly hungry, overweight, and drained of any kind of energy. A lot of people think that they will feel bad if they eat less frequently. Maybe for the first few days that's true. But give it a couple weeks. With Intermittent Fasting I have boundless energy. I had no idea of the physical potential I've had hiding within until now.
Jessica from Los Angeles	Don't be afraid! It's not hard at all and you're going to love how you feel when fasting. You can enjoy life, reap some health benefits, and lose weight. You'll wish you had started earlier!
Patti from KY	I wish I knew not to panic the first time I got hungry before it was time to eat and feel like I had failed. As time went on, I learned what hunger really meant and if really hungry then I eat.
Ginger P from Florida	It is OK to start with slow fast and then build up to bigger ones. This is a brand new philosophy and it can be easy to want to jump in too fast and do long windows of fasting. Remember that you did not get here overnight and it can be a safe bet that this new lifestyle will take time. Trust the process and trust your body. Start wherever you can and build up from there!

cont.

Ally Pski	I wish I would have known that this is not an impossible dream like all of the other plans I have tried. This really does become a comfortable way of life and you will lose weight somewhat effortlessly. The mental part of your food relationship will exist and will need to be worked through, especially as you start seeing changes happening. It feels almost unreal to be successful without all of the work that the other plans had, like you are doing something wrong. Trust in the process, be kind to yourself, and enjoy a life of successes you never knew you needed.
Michele Singletary	Hunger is not an emergency. I wish I had known that I would not die or even come close to death by skipping a meal . . . or 2 . . . or 3 or 4. I could not fathom it would be so effortless to miss a meal but feel so great. This is what I hear the most when telling folks about IF. The response is often "I have to eat first thing in the morning. I can't skip meals . . . I will feel bad if I do." If only I had known . . . hunger is not an emergency.
MaryKHN	I wish I had known about IF years ago—I wish I had known how easy it was to lose weight and gain health using this method. I heard about IF and started doing it the same day. My life would be different if I had known about this years ago. I wish I had known that it would clear up the headaches I have had since childhood (I'm now 59 and have dealt with cluster and migraine headaches for 50+ years), that it would clear up my ezcema that I have had since I was 4 or 5, that my joint pain would go away, that my skin would appear smoother and younger. This is the most amazing way of life.
Andy Hanson	I wish I knew that almost everything I'd been told about weight gain, diet, and exercise was wrong. At 46 years old, I've been obese since I got out of the Marine Corps 21 years ago. I thought it was because I wasn't eating right and wasn't moving enough. The problem is, dads who work desk jobs and eat three square meals a day plus snacks while exercising an hour a day WILL gain weight. I wish I knew because I used to beat myself up daily for being a failure while actually making so-called "healthy" lifestyle choices. I wish I knew that common sense is actually right—eating less frequently will make you lose weight. Eating makes you fat. Not eating makes you not fat. I wish I knew how easy it is to go 18-24 hours without eating, and that doing so wouldn't destroy my metabolism. Sometimes I feel like I've hurt my body for years because I was doing what I was supposed to do, and it makes me upset. Then, I realize that I have a lot to be thankful for. I HAD high blood pressure and cholesterol, now after a little over three months of eating one meal a day, my cholesterol is normal. I'm thankful that I learned about IF before being diagnosed with diabetes, as my mother and many of my aunts and uncles have. I'm thankful that using keto I dropped from 270 to 242, and in three months of eating one meal a day, I'm down to 220. I'm thankful that now when I go for a walk I feel the NEED to run. I used to hate running, now my legs are screaming for me to move them faster.
Diane K.	What I wish I knew when I first started IF is how easy it would be to make this a way of life forever!

Angie Stark	I wish that I had known that IF is not starvation—that I would not feel weak or light-headed, but rather, that my body would operate so much better with this way of eating. I knew of 2 people with very different background/ lifestyles, etc. who had success with IF, but I automatically dismissed it as something that I could never do, or that could not work for me. I lumped it in with every other "diet" fad. Boy, was I wrong!
Kathleen DDS	Often trying every possible diet, pill, excercise program, food timing strategies, healthy eating, etc you name it I tried it. Years of eating foods that sometimes I wanted to gag, stressing to feed my body every 3 hours because "that's the only way you can increase your metabolism" . . . NOT! Deprivation to the point I was very cranky, then of course watching the scale drop down VERY very slowly only to see it go back up 10 times quicker than the weeks and months it took for it to go down. I am now 61 years young and for the first time in my life I can live a daily life NEVER feeling deprived as I follow a true Delay DON'T Deny philosophy. If I only would have known that fasting and not depriving myself would make me look and feel better than I have in years! If I would have known about the science of IF years ago I would not have spent so much money over the years on many diet books, diet pills and different sizes in clothes! Would not have missed out on many special occasions cause I was avoiding events due to how I looked or what food/ drink I had to avoid. Better late than NEVER! A true lifestyle change not a diet. Even on a day I celebrate with a longer window or more treats or cocktails, I no longer ever feel guilty!
Jen L.	I wish I didn't hesitate in starting IF for as long as I did. I was nervous about the possibility of failure but intermittent fasting has been the best, easiest change I could have possibly made to my life. With all the dietary standards we've been fed for years, it's hard to believe I could be so energized without eating small frequent meals. I love how easy my life has become. Don't hesitate to give it a try!
Rania	I have struggled with losing weight for a long time but with IF there is no struggle. You MUST clean fast and ditch the scale and you have to give it some time, be patient and I promise you will see results. I have lost 59 pounds in 11 months, I just trusted the process and kept it moving. I am so happy with the results and the transformation I have made. Just do it and don't look back!!!
Debbie Pisciotta	1. I wish I knew about intermittent fasting 30 years ago. 2. I wish I knew that your body doesn't need 3 meals a day plus snacks to to be healthy. 3. I wish I knew that intermittent fasting can help reverse type 2 diabetes since it runs in my family. 4. I wish I knew about the clean fast. I used to drink diet soda and diet iced tea to fill me up and only made it harder. Once I clean fasted it was so much easier and intermittent fasting became the easiest thing I have ever done. IF rocks!

cont.

Leah Jo	I started doing Intermittent Fasting before I read *Delay Don't Deny* so I didn't recognize how important the clean fast was and someone had told me I could have cream in my coffee. What a difference it made when I found Gin's strict guidelines on clean fasting, with the science to back it up. It makes so much sense and made the world of difference for my fasting. I came to Intermittent Fasting for the health benefits, but have also seen a reduction in weight and that stubborn fat around the middle. Now that I clean fast I am keeping IF as a way of life!
Lisa H from New Hampshire	Trust the process, internal healing takes time. Change up your fasting windows once in a while when you plateau. Don't be hard on yourself, start fresh everyday.
Andrea from Indianapolis	Before I began IF, I wish I knew it was vital to 100% clean fast. In my window, feast doesn't mean total abandon. Until I got a grasp on those concepts I wasn't getting all the benefits.
Nicole A	No matter what I read in the book or on the online support group pages I couldn't fathom the idea of going that long without eating. I figured these must be some kind of "super people" with incredible strength. I know I'm strong but was I that strong? Well, turns out you don't need a super power to do this. After the first couple of days it got easier and easier and my fasting time started increasing almost by accident. Soon I could do 40 hours no problem. Long story short, I wish I knew how easy this lifestyle is despite your inner voice thinking it's beyond comprehension or doable.
Shana Smith	I remember being at my "maximum capacity" or highest weight and thinking "if I could just lose 20 pounds I'd be SO much happier!" Then it happened . . . after 3 months I lost 20 pounds! I was very happy BUT when the weight loss stagnated my spirits dipped. Thankfully I had taken pictures AND measurements of my body from the beginning. I tried on the same dress and snapped a selfie. Wow! I could see how much my stomach had shrunk. When the scale refused to move or lied because of hormone flux, I could turn to the measuring tape and see change there. I realized that taking more weight off would be a long-term plan, but that it was easy to keep the 20 lbs. or more off once it was finally lost! The pictures and measurements reminded me how far I had come and that I wasn't going back.
Mo Cannon	Wish I learned this way of L*IF*E sooner. This is the easiest thing I have ever done in trying to reach my healthy goal weight. Listen to your body, it will tell you when you NEED to eat, and often what you need to eat. Take it one day and even one meal at a time. YOU CAN DO THIS!
Net M.	Give IF one full month of commitment before you even begin to think it doesn't work for you. It took me that much time to really get comfortable with the process and to completely 'clean' fast. Give IF 3 months to fine tune your fasting and feasting schedule and to really begin to feel the benefits in store for you. Give IF 4-6 months to see the inches really begin to come off.

	Don't make the process harder than it actually is. AND . . . . .Yes, it WORKS. I always crave what is forbidden to me. That is why Delay, Don't Deny Intermittent Fasting works for me: no forbidden food.
Lisa Wooley	You WILL eventually develop a "Fasting Muscle" allowing you to go all day without needing food. The hunger is so bad in the beginning that you are ravenous when you hit that kitchen door at night!! After time this extreme feeling isn't there; you'll be able to casually prepare dinner even if it takes a while. It's freedom from all the diet rules . . .
Julie from Augusta	I spent so many years trying to eat "correct" foods three times a day. It was so hard to figure out what the rules were. I was desperate for a plan I could live with long term. I had no idea that not eating was actually a choice and was the answer I was searching for. Once I bought into the importance of the clean fast, IF became so easy for me mentally. I can never see myself eating any other way.
Roxi	What I wish I knew before starting IF is that I wasn't to blame for my weight. I had done all the things I was told to do . . . exercised 7 times a week, ate 4 to 5 small meals a day, etc. It was never about calories in/calories out. It was about hormones and the timing of our food. I really wish that's what I had known all along because the guilt people have can feel like a life sentence. And no one should have to feel that way.
Megan Flanagan	The best thing about IF is the flexibility. Some days I eat a ton, some days I'm satisfied after one meal, some days I go for a short 13-hour fast, most days I fast for 16 hours or more. I had a bad day a week into IF where I gorged myself and ate into the wee hours. That would've been enough to completely give up on any diet I've tried, but IF is not a diet, it's a way of life, and tomorrow's a new day. This week I completed my first 20-hour fast and I feel great!
Loretta	We hear it again and again but it's so true. We are each an N of 1 in this experience. Gather data (weight and measurements), evaluate progress, tweak and fast on!
Ann Handy	I wish I knew about IF before I did all of these crazy diets, and spent so much money !!! I am so amazed at how this way of life has changed me. I can feel my hips, and my face and body do not feel bloated. I mainly do a 20:4 with one meal a day, and at 54 people are telling me I look so much younger. I have adopted and embraced this lifestyle of health and couldn't be more satisfied and look forward to what comes next!
Jaya Navy Wife	Don't deny anything, and soon you won't want to eat everything!
Girl with an Indiana Appetite	IF truly is a mind-set. It's not easy, but nothing of value in life is easy. Personally, I like to look at fasting time as a challenge, because I can feel proud of myself when it's done. Don't think about what you CANNOT eat, think about when you can eat! Nothing is off the table, but your choices

cont.

	WILL change for the better & you will look back shortly and be so grateful that you rose to the challenge. Also, ditch the scale . . . more than once it has caused doubt and anxiety that I did not need. More than anything else, it made me question the success of this lifestyle. Never again . . .
Kimberly Colarossi	Research! Learn! Google! Podcast! Join support groups! Seeing results and hearing the stories of real-life people and struggles makes it real! My husband said it's not healthy to eat once a day. I researched. It is!! I am a breast cancer survivor and to learn my cells can rejuvenate while fasting is amazing! I thought how can I not eat for 20 hours?? This isn't going to be good. Well I did! For the first 2 days I had a slight headache but not bad. When I opened my window I was shocked at how full I was fast! I felt great! I'm not obese but at 5'4" and 55 years old I just looked at food and the weight came on. I found myself not able to lose but gain no matter what I tried. I saw a Facebook friend started the IF journey and 12 lbs. in 1 week were lost! I needed to know more. She said buy Gin's book! It makes sense! So I jumped in headfirst and starting fasting and then bought the book! It's an eye-opener! I do one meal a day within 20:4 and have never felt better. I've lost weight from 164 to 158 in one week. I see the belly fat shifting. I see my clothes fit a bit better. I feel amazing and I'm eating healthy but what I want to eat. Wine included!!! When you can eat Chicago deep dish pizza for break-fast and lose weight and feel great . . . that's a great thing! I also move my window to fit my lifestyle. I don't sacrifice lifestyle for fasting! That was important! IF is not a lifestyle it's my new way of life!!!! My advice to my friends is give it a try . . . you might just be surprised! I'm a skeptic to a believer!!! Living a healthy no-diet way of life! Thank you Gin!!!
Mary Moffit	IF is the way to escape from dieting. ANY other plan you can choose WILL restrict you from something you love. If you struggle with chronic dieting then you know you will eventually fail. Nothing is off-limits with IF! Remind yourself it's just "not now" versus "not ever." Want ice cream? Great! Have it at 7pm. The food freedom is life-changing.
Tracy Bratton	IF is a process and a lifestyle change; not a diet. You must be willing to have patience and grace with yourself and your body. Healing takes time. Do NOT compare yourself to others and know that you will need to try various eating patterns, lengths of fast, and eating windows. Enjoy the journey!
Andrea McGary	I wish I knew that IF was actually a beautiful journey in freedom. Freedom from all the diet rules I followed for far too long. I was in chains. IF has given me the freedom to enjoy butter and cheese with pure delight. IF has given me the freedom to trust my body. I am free, and it feels so good.
Jenny	I wish I knew that weight doesn't automatically fall right off in the beginning. I wish I had known about the clean fast from the beginning. I wasn't clean fasting for quite a while. I wish I knew I didn't need to be afraid to weigh myself. I have avoided going to the doctor for YEARS because I didn't want to know what I

	weighed. I have been weighing myself daily for over a month and it's been interesting to see the daily fluctuations. (I know this isn't for everyone but it has helped me.)
Kathy Wheeler	When I started intermittent fasting, the long-embedded diet mentality had me convinced that I still had to count calories, and that carbs and fat were bad. In essence, I was back on yet another diet AND intermittent fasting—oh joy! I knew then that the diet mentality had to go and that IF would be the key to loss and sustainable maintenance. The other important bit of advice I would give is to stay curious about the why, what and how of intermittent fasting. I've never wanted to know more about what I was doing to get healthy before, as long as the scale would drop . . . and FAST, I'd do anything (and we all know how that turns out)! With intermittent fasting, the more I learn from experts and others' experiences, the more I know this is the right path because it all makes sense. One last thing, do yourself a favor—don't compare your journey to anyone else's. If you understand the why, what and how, you'll be okay with however your journey progresses.
Susie L	I wish I knew that I would feel so good and that it's so much easier than I expected! All the years of diets and diet books that were nothing more than a temporary fix. The very best thing is that I'm able to cook as I finally wish. Healthy foods for sure, but recipes are now unlimited. Things that I wanted to make but felt I couldn't because I was on another diet. Holidays aren't scary. No guilt to enjoy the day. I adjust the fasting to fit my schedule. Ahhhh FREEDOM!
Tracy from Santa Barbara	You have to trust the process. For some people, the body releases fat quickly, for others it is slower. Remind yourself as often as needed "Hunger is not an emergency." Slow everything down. Make food choices slowly and thoughtfully. Eat slowly. Stop eating when you are no longer hungry. Pause and then if you're still hungry thirty minutes later have something else. I promise you, you won't expire if you don't eat for 16, 18, 20+ hours. Drink water. Get to know what it feels like to feel "empty." It is so freeing. Understand that you are making a life decision, not a food decision, not a diet for now decision but a decision about how you can live with freedom for the rest of your life. WHAT YOU WEIGH DOES NOT DEFINE YOU. Your body adjusts and becomes the powerful source of energy and vibrancy and clarity that it was meant to be. All of that is WAY more important than a number on a scale. You are WORTH IT. What else are you going to do? Research, test foods, eat a variety of food. Tweak. Tweak. Tweak. There is NO PERFECT, there is just freedom. We're here to help. :)
Sue Werley	I wish I knew the physiological aspects of fasting. For much of my overweight life I had been encouraged to eat three meals and three snacks per day. And to "track" that food. It was exhausting. And, even if you stayed within the "program," you may lose four OUNCES a week. How hard that was. I felt like such a failure.

cont.

	Now, I fast between 18-20 hours each day. I still am careful about what and how much I eat, but that is more in relation to what my body needs for fuel. I am wearing clothes that I haven't worn for years and I haven't weighed myself for over a month.
Laurel Wilson	When my husband first explained IF to me I thought he was crazy. After he explained the science behind it, I thought I might as well give it a shot. I then attacked every book, lecture, interview and podcast I could find. As a person that has struggled with weight since puberty, it has been nothing short of amazing. I feel in control of my eating and at peace around food. One of the best things about it is the flexibility it gives you to live the lifestyle. Vegan? Paleo? Breakfast eater? No problem! Although it sounds very challenging, most people I have talked to comment that it isn't as challenging as it sounds. I used to mourn that I was such a food addict. I felt it was impossible to eat 4-5 times a day—day after day—and keep it reasonable. Often people who are addicted to cigarettes, alcohol or other things go cold turkey and swear off the substance that is so damaging to their health. I longed for a similar solution to my situation. Turns out IF was that solution I was seeking.
Janet K Price	I wish I would've known that it worked, that a clean fast is the ONLY way to FAST and that your body could repair and heal itself through FASTING.
Vicki Jamison	Weight control is less about willpower and more about the science of eating. I believed for all of my adult life that I had no willpower to control my eating. Just a couple of months of not eating breakfast and clean fasts and I found myself being able to pass up sweets that sat on my counter. A couple more months of IF and OMAD and I found I would come to a point in my eating where I just couldn't eat another bite, previously unknown behavior for me. A couple more months and I found that I was spending less and less time thinking about eating and more time just living and staying busy. I just wish I had understood for all those years that eating made me hungry.
Cynthia Eike	I wish I had known that my instinct about eating 5 or 6 times a day was sabotaging me! I hated being a slave to snacks and small meals. This is the most freeing way of life ever!
Kate from Atlanta	This is not about being perfect—it's about a journey. Know your motivation—know your "why" but ultimately know that opening your window isn't a failure but a learning . . . understand "why" and accept. Adjust and grow. I no longer feel like I am failing if I eat more calories or points. I focus on how I am feeling to move to success.
Lindsey Bell	Hunger is not a constant state; it will come and go if you push through it. I've actually learned to enjoy my brief feelings of hunger because I imagine that my body is using my reserved food supply (body fat) to fuel itself!

	Some people are able to eat whatever they want during their window. I've experimented enough with my own eating habits to know that's not the case for me. If I make an effort to eat whole foods, I feel better and tend to lose more weight. If I eat processed carbs, I find it harder to fast the next day because I crave more carbs. Do your own experiments and find out what works for YOU!
Amy from Knoxville	I wish I knew how easy IF would get in a short amount of time AND that clean fasting makes all the difference in the world. I couldn't make it much past 14 hours when fasting drinking cream in my coffee. Since starting up again this summer, I clean fast and within 3-4 weeks black coffee is wonderful and it's nothing to look at the clock and it's been 18-19 hours. It truly becomes a way of life!
Kristi Taylor	I wish I would have known about IF 30 years ago. It has caused me to throw away so much misinformation that was "programmed" in my brain for so long. Simple, supportive, and not even a diet. It's a lifestyle, a very sustainable lifestyle. I remember my grandmother used to encourage everyone to stop eating at sundown and begin again at sun up. It makes so much sense now!
Beach Lover Kim	I wish I better understood the freedom I would gain by just foregoing a few meals and snacks per day! Freedom from having to join the post-menopausal "weight gain club" and that "inevitable" belly fat. Freedom from skin tags, rough elbows and dry skin. Freedom from hypercholesterolemia, pre-diabetes and metabolic syndrome. Freedom to enjoy life on my own terms and freedom to have a positive impact on my future. Freedom to be the best wife, mother, and grandmother into the future. You won't REALLY know these things without taking that first step and giving it your best try. Not always easy—but worth it!
Denise from Wisconsin	Starting with an 8-hour eating window and working gradually down to a 5-hour window over a few weeks made adopting an intermittent fasting lifestyle surprisingly easy. My first week I also gave myself permission to take it really easy, like I was on a personal wellness retreat. My IF motivation was to reduce inflammation due to arthritis and that happened by the fourth week! No more aspirin every 4 hours to get through the day. After 3 months of IF with clean fasting I also had the extra bonus of a 20 lb. weight loss. Yay! IF for LIFE!
Paula Praline from Baton Rouge	I first bought the book *Delay Don't Deny* back in April 2018. After reading it I thought no way I can do this. I was convinced after decades of dieting, I needed to eat early breakfast. I was incredibly hungry all the time. I joined the DDD online support group. Seeing all the success stories and hearing people talk about their appetite correction, I had hope this could work so I hopped on board. It's been amazing. I'm no longer hungry all the time. My food obsession is gone and I'm smaller than I have been in many years. But what's more amazing are the results of my 20-year-old daughter. She was diagnosed with PCOS in her early teens and has never

cont.

	had normal consecutive cycles. She saw the results I was having and decided to join me. She has lost 20 pounds and is super fit. She recently went back to the endocrinologist and asked him if she could stop the birth control to see if she'd have a natural cycle. He told her yes she could try to stop the pills but he felt with the particular type of PCOS she has, that natural occurring cycle would not happen. Well guess what, she's had two normal cycles. To me this is huge for many reasons. This is an answered prayer.
Joy from Texas	What I wish I knew is how helpful it is to become aware of what meaning I give to fasting and eating. Fasting is not punishment. Eating is not reward. If the meaning I give to fasting is to "make up for" anything, that baggage of regret complicates the simplicity of "window open" and "window closed." My past choices are behind me. I have this moment to set my fasting window and get on with my life until the time I choose to open my eating window. Rewriting the meaning I give to both fasting and eating as both health investment and self-care has made my multiple year maintenance successful. Old meanings can creep back in for me, at which time, my pants typically get tighter. I do revisit the past when I see old patterns sneaking in, but only to examine meanings like a kind detective who makes no judgement calls. Typically, the question is "what meaning did I give to that (meal, fasting window, food item, etc)?" Followed by, "was that meaning true and beneficial? What do I truly need to take care of myself?" Finishing with an affirmation, "what is true is that fasting is a healthy way to take care of myself, and eating is a healthy way to nourish myself enjoyably. I am learning better self-care with kindness and gentleness with myself."
Pam	Don't expect to immediately lose weight. Based on past dieting experiences, it seems that weight would just fall off if you are fasting, but it doesn't necessarily. And this is very frustrating and confusing if you are not mentally prepared for this. How can you be so hungry at first, and not lose a pound? Patience pays off.
Lucy Mars	After the first few weeks, it became so easy to spend my day on other activities and to not have to stop for food or even think about eating, even when I was teaching cookery. I also hadn't even realized that I restricted myself in what I ate & judged myself for eating 'too much cheese' or putting butter on my potatoes. With IF, I freely eat whatever I really want, and as much as I want, every single day. It's fantastic! I never have to 'make up for' an indulgent meal, by restricting myself the following day. I can also eat out with gusto! Some days I'm not very hungry, so I eat very little, and that's fine too, but I can still eat whatever I want and relish every mouthful.
Sarah from College Station, TX	I wish I knew what "Trust the process" meant. With all the crazy diets out there, we are so conditioned to wanting to see results the second we eat 10 calories less than normal. Because I loved the idea of not eating all the time, I stuck with it even though I didn't lose weight for the first month and am so glad I did.

	The best advice for a new Intermittent Faster is start slow (don't jump to ADF), let your body grieve not getting food every hour, be okay with no or little weight loss at first, and stick with it for the long haul. You will be so glad you did!
Emily Sanders	I wish I knew that I would not be hungry during the fasting period. I've been pleasantly surprised that I feel so good while drinking just water while fasting. I wish I knew that I could eat what I want without measuring food, counting calories, tracking food, etc. I wish I knew that my arthritis pain would disappear. I wish I knew that it would be so easy. I had tried many weight loss plans and always felt hungry . . . or frustrated . . . or depleted financially. I wish I knew that I would feel younger and more fit, as a result of IF. I wish I knew that I would not be dizzy or faint while fasting. I wish I knew that the anti-inflammatory benefits were so immediate. I felt a noticeable difference—in a positive way—within the first week of intermittent fasting! Don't be afraid to try this! It gave me a new lease on life and a renewed sense of hope for developing a healthy lifestyle.
Pam from TX	DELAY is the key word . . . I have not DENIED anything, and have lost over 30 lb in a year. . . . .because it's NOT a diet, it's a Way Of Life (WOL). DIET=unsustainable weight loss. I am happy to lose slowly because I know I can KEEP it off! And because it's a Way of Life, I can adjust/modify my eating patterns to fit my life. . . . vacations, holidays, etc. with NO GUILT!!! When could you do THAT on a DIET??? Thank you, Gin.
Laine Irvine from beautiful NZ	Take one day at a time and you don't have to be perfect in your eating window. Just be sure to have a clean fast.
Emma D	Wish I'd known that everyone's journey is different. Don't compare yourself to others. I took 2.5 months to get more energy and over two months to become fat-adapted. And it was worth the wait!
Franki from Adelaide	To be patient. Just as it took time to get into bad habits, good habits take time to kick in but boy, once it does! I will NEVER eat like I used to again. Believe in the process and the testimonies of success. Use online support groups to learn from fellow IFs. I'm 61 next year and healthiest I have ever been. It works!
Michelle from Sydney	I'm just amazed at how much IF has helped with my back pain. I just move around so much more easily now since I started fasting. It has also helped me be in control of my eating rather than feeling out of control. I feel much more disciplined. Wish I had started IF years ago.
Caitlyn Carraher	I wish I knew how much energy I would have. I have started to dance around my house just because I have all this excess energy that needs an outlet. I wake up refreshed. No fog or grogginess. I drink coffee because I enjoy it, not for the energy boost and have switched to decaf for my second cup of the day.

cont.

Lesley from Australia	I wish I knew how good I'd feel and how effortless this way of life is. Start easy, just push back your breakfast to 10am then 11am; before you know it you're at 2pm or 3pm and you're easily eating later, fasting longer and feeling G-R-E-A-T.
Sara Bauer	Intermittent fasting brings a peace and clarity to your life you may not have known was missing. Finding you have it in you to do this powerful thing, taking control of your body, will give you confidence and power to take control of the other important aspects of your life. Have you always wished you could accomplish something great? You can! You will. And you can do it again and again. You will find this out.
Claudette Gosselin Mullen	Concentrate on how you are feeling leading an IF lifestyle, celebrate, and I mean in a *BIG* way, all the non-scale victories along the way, because this, and not weight loss, has made it my life changing way of life!!! And the #1 thing that I wish I understood on day 1 was it IS a process/progression that you must go through, so remember to observe each change and most of all CELEBRATE, it makes life SO much easier and you truly are SO much happier than before IF. "Delay, Don't Deny" is a daily mantra!
Diane from St. Louis	I WISH I had known about, read about, or heard about IF so many YEARS ago. Imagine if this amazing IF information was a widespread method, life lesson, similar to "cigarettes are bad for you" for the last 20 or more years. The weight & health of a nation, and ME, could be so, so much better. I wish I had known how easy it is to DELAY!!!
Sarah from Ashland	I wish I knew that the old feeling I would get when I went a long time without eating is NOT the same as how you feel when your body is a trained "faster." Now, I do get hungry, but I never get "hangry." I never get that low blood sugar, jittery, uncomfortable panicky feeling. I just get hunger pangs, which go away, and I get NO other physical symptoms. I was a person who believed I was incapable of going a long time without eating. I felt terrible. Now I am a total convert. I eat dinner and sometimes a small snack in midafternoon. I had no idea I was not only capable of this, but that it would actually feel physically better to do it this way.
Ceci	As a nurse, my brain initially rebelled. Time restricted eating seemed so counterintuitive. But like many things in life, allowing yourself to question your "truths" can open up a whole new world of possibilities. It can be freeing. I have a couple of autoimmune diseases that have significantly improved. Yes, from time to time you will experience hunger, especially at first, but hunger pangs are fleeting. I often think about the many on our planet who go to bed hungry every single day. I think of the parents who have no idea how they will feed their children. I've become more grateful for my abundance. I choose more carefully and I eat more mindfully.

Ginny from Woodstock	I was tired of thinking about food literally ALL DAY when I decided to try IF. All of the information was very helpful, and helped me to decide that this way of life would be for me. What I didn't know was that I would really begin to ENJOY food again. For years I've weighed, measured, counted everything I ate. Now I'm mindful, but I don't obsess about the tracking of each ingredient I'm putting in my mouth. It's so freeing. It also makes cooking less of a chore. I'm not tracking/weighing, figuring out the calorie/carb count for each serving. I cook with quality ingredients, and let myself eat until I'm full and satisfied.
Tammy Haldeman	I wish I knew how valuable the information and advice I got before I started really was. I had a very very close friend who fasted before me. I was one of the lucky ones. I was given all the answers, but I didn't know how valuable the advice really was. 1. Trust the process isn't just a phrase. If you do the clean fast and you fast every day and you commit to your hours and your window it works —for health and for weight loss. 2. It's not a matter of if IF will work for you, it's a matter of how and when. Everyone is different and an experiment of one. 3. Trust yourself and your body to do what it needs. Eat what is good for YOU and your body will tell you what is not working. 4. Make your window a vault! When it's closed nothing gets in except coffee and water. It can't. It's closed. 5. Hunger isn't an emergency. It won't kill you. It's temporary. Pretend you are somewhere with no food and push through.
Lindsey K.	I've realized sugar really is THE WORST for me. I don't deny sugar entirely, but I'm way more conscious of it and the way it makes me feel. I'm so much less bloated (reduced inflammation), and even my mood is so much more stable and elevated. I used to sip sugar-free drinks all day, thinking I was being "healthy," but now I realize I was just confusing my hormones all day. Our bodies are not as evolved as we'd like to think . . . Our culture and food availability has shifted rapidly and significantly over the last century. We should really strive to eat as our grandparents and great-grandparents did: mostly homemade, "real" food, one large meal a day, unsweetened drinks to hydrate. Having one primary meal a day allows me to focus on quality and gives me freedom the rest of the day. I'm saving time and money while losing weight and improving my health!
Amanda from Baltimore	First, it gets easier. Day by day, bit by bit, even if you only extend your fasting window by 15 minutes, you can get there. Second, everyone's journey is different. Don't get caught up in other people's success stories who lost 100 lbs. doing 16:8 and could eat whatever they wanted to. Our bodies are all different. Third, read about the science and take strangers' advice with a grain of salt. Not everyone on the internet is an expert.

cont.

	Finally, this is a lifestyle and not a diet. For me it's about getting my body to function the way it was intended to and not so much about weight loss. There is some give and take to find what makes my body happiest. However, that does not mean IF will cure all your ailments, it just means I'm not a slave to food and my body can function better if I'm not constantly eating.
IF'er from Surrey UK	Living a DDD lifestyle is the best thing you can do for your health. Weight loss may be slow to start with because the body prioritizes internal healing over weight loss. But once that is dealt with it's amazing how the body can give up fat and gain muscle. Two years down the line, I am now the slimmest I have been since my early 20s.

FREQUENTLY ASKED QUESTIONS

WHO SHOULD FAST, AND WHO SHOULD NOT FAST?

GENERAL QUESTIONS

- What if I get hungry during the fast? (p. 280)

- How should I handle social situations that occur when my eating window is closed? On a related note, how should I handle pressure to eat when I don't want to eat? (p. 281)

- Is it better to track my fasting hours or to track my eating window? (p. 283)

- What if my fasting / eating window times don't add up to twenty-four? (p. 284)

- Can I do a twenty-four-hour fast every day? (p. 285)

- If fasting is so healthy, why don't I just fast for days/weeks/months until I get to my goal weight? (p. 285)

- Can I split up my day into TWO eating windows? Meaning, have breakfast from 8:00 a.m. to 9:00 a.m., close my window, fast until dinner, and then eat from 6:00 p.m. to 7:00 p.m.? (p. 286)

- My window is closing, and I'm not hungry. Should I eat more food now so I won't be hungry later? (p. 286)

- I already closed my window for the day, but I am STARVING. What should I do? (p. 286)

- Help! I accidentally tasted food / sipped a non-fast-compliant beverage during the fast. What do I do? (p. 286)

- Can I / should I have a "cheat" day? (p. 287)

- How do I explain what I am doing to my children? (p. 287)

CAN I HAVE ___ WHILE FASTING?

- Will I still lose weight if I don't follow the recommendations for a clean fast? (p. 288)

- I saw a video that said it's okay to have _____ while fasting, but you say it isn't okay. Why is there disagreement about what to have while fasting? (p. 289)

- I heard an expert say that coffee and tea break the fast, and we should stick to water only. What's up with that? (p. 290)

- What should I do about my medications and supplements? Do they break the fast? (p. 290)

- I have to take a daily medication with food, and the recommended dosage times fall within my fasting time. What should I do? (p. 291)

- How do I know if _____ is okay to have during the fast? (p. 291)

- Does Communion break the fast? (p. 292)

- Does vaping / chewing tobacco / smoking break the fast? (p. 292)

- Can I take exogenous ketones while fasting? (p. 293)

- What can I have during the fast to combat bad breath? (p. 294)

- Can I use flavored lip balm during the fast? (p. 294)

- Can I take a fiber supplement during the fast? (p. 295)

FOOD CHOICES / NUTRITION

- What is the best thing to eat when I open my eating window? (p. 295)

- Should I count calories / carbs / fat / and so on during my eating window just to be sure that I don't overeat? (p. 296)

- How can I make sure to get in all my daily calories with a shorter eating window? (p. 296)

- Why am I bingeing as soon as I open my eating window? (p. 296)

- Do I need to worry about not getting enough nutrients since I'm eating less food? (p. 297)

MEDICAL QUESTIONS

- I feel shaky/nauseous during the fast. What should I do? (p. 297)

- Can I do IF with a medical condition? (p. 297)

- Will IF heal my medical condition? (p. 298)

- Why do I have constipation/diarrhea now that I have started IF? (p. 298)

- I have noticed that I am losing my hair. What's going on? Is this common? (p. 299)

- My doctor has never heard of intermittent fasting / says intermittent fasting only works because you reduce calories / says that intermittent fasting will slow my metabolism, and so on. Why doesn't my doctor know the current research on IF, and what can I do? (p. 299)

- Is IF helpful for someone with PCOS? (p. 300)

EXERCISE

- What is the best time of day to work out? (p. 300)

- My trainer told me that I had to have protein immediately before/after/during my workout. Is that true? And I'm worried that I am not getting in enough protein during my eating window. Don't I need to eat a lot of protein to build muscle? (p. 300)

- Can I take a pre-workout/post-workout/BCAAs/other exercise supplements during the fast? (p. 301)

TRACKING YOUR PROGRESS

- Will I lose _____ pounds in _____ days/weeks/months? (p. 301)

- Why am I losing clothing sizes but no pounds on the scale? (p. 302)

PHYSIOLOGY OF FASTING

- Help! I can't sleep. What can I do? (p. 308)

- Why does my blood sugar go up during the fast? (p. 308)

- Why is my cholesterol higher now than before I started IF? (p. 308)

WHO SHOULD FAST, AND WHO SHOULD NOT FAST?

Is it safe for children or teens to fast?

As I mentioned in chapter 9, please do not put your children onto an intermittent fasting regimen, even if you are concerned that they are over-weight. Refer to that chapter for more information. If you have teenagers, check with your child's physician to see if and when IF may be right for them.

Can someone with type 1 diabetes fast?

This is a conversation to have with your doctor. Type 1 diabetics produce no (or very little) insulin on their own, so it's essential to monitor blood glucose as directed to make sure levels remain in a safe range. Because intermittent fasters are not eating regularly, insulin needs will be different from when following a more typical eating pattern.

Can someone with type 2 diabetes fast?

Scientific research into the effects of intermittent fasting on those with type 2 diabetes is promising.[1] Dr. Jason Fung, author of *The Diabetes Code*, reports that many of his patients have reversed their type 2 diabetes through intermittent fasting, dietary changes, or a combination of both. In fact, he and colleagues released a short case study article in 2018 in which they reported the effectiveness of intermittent fasting as a tool to reverse type 2 diabetes.[2] If you or someone you love has type 2 diabetes (or is prediabetic), I highly recommend starting with Dr. Fung's book. As always, discuss your plans with your own doctor/endocrinologist to make sure it is right for you.

Is it safe for women to do IF? I read a blog post / heard from a friend / watched a video that said that women shouldn't do IF or that women need to do IF in a special way. And will IF affect my menstrual cycle?

If you ask Uncle Google, you can find all sorts of cautionary blog posts and videos expressing concern and debating whether women are just too delicate for intermittent fasting. Remember, though—in the not-too-distant past, women were also considered too delicate for running, voting, and wearing pants.

It's true that women's bodies are different from men's bodies, and it's also true that we don't respond well to long-term over-dieting or over-restriction. Yep. Truth. But! All throughout this book, I have cautioned you (whether you are male *or* female) to avoid over-dieting and over-restriction. That's important for *all* of us, no matter our gender. So, ladies, don't over-diet and over-restrict, and also don't couple that type of behavior with an intense workout regimen. (Men, you also shouldn't do that.) If you start to feel like you may be overdoing it, you're probably right. In that case, scale it back a little (or scale it back a lot) until you feel great again. Never forget that sometimes less is more.

What does the research say? One 2016 study found that a seventy-two-hour fast did not affect the menstrual cycle of normal cycling women.[3] A 2016 literature review that examined all the available research related to women and fasting found that fasting has actually been linked to an *improvement* in women's reproductive health.[4] Overall, they concluded that "fasting can be prescribed as a safe medical intervention as well as a lifestyle regimen which can improve women's health in many folds." I'll trust these scientists over an internet blog or scary video.

One thing women do need to know—when you first start IF, you may actually experience changes in your menstrual cycle for a few months. If you're nervous and want confirmation that this is normal, search for a blog post written by Megan Ramos, who has experience guiding thousands of women through medically supervised fasting protocols under the direction of Dr. Jason Fung in the Intensive Dietary Management clinic. Her blog post is called "Women and Fasting: Does Fasting Affect Your Cycle," and she explains what you should expect as your body adjusts to IF. She describes how cycle disruptions are common at first but that their patients' bodies generally adapt and begin running like clockwork after a few months. Of course, if you are concerned, check with your own doctor for advice.

Is it safe to fast while pregnant or trying to conceive?

As I mentioned in chapter 9, fasting is not recommended for women who are pregnant. Refer to that chapter for more information.

The question becomes more difficult to answer if you are trying to conceive. Certain medical conditions related to infertility, such as PCOS (polycystic ovary syndrome) may actually benefit from intermittent fasting, and in our IF support groups, we have seen numerous PCOS sufferers announce their pregnancies after living an IF lifestyle for a while. See the Medical Questions section of the FAQ for more information about PCOS and fasting.

If you're trying to conceive and are concerned about whether IF is right for you, I recommend talking to your ob-gyn just to be on the safe side.

Is fasting safe for breastfeeding mothers?

As I mentioned in chapter 9, fasting is not recommended for women who are breastfeeding. Refer to that chapter for more information.

Can fasting lead to the development of eating disorders?

As I mentioned in chapter 9, fasting is not recommended for anyone with a diagnosed eating disorder. Refer to that chapter for more information.

It's important to note that fasting itself will not cause an eating disorder but that someone with an eating disorder may find that fasting triggers the disordered behavior. If you ever become concerned, please speak to a medical professional or a counselor trained in working with eating disorders.

Can I / should I fast when I am ill?

My go-to answer to this question is that you should always listen to your body when you are sick. If you think eating would make you feel better, eat. If you think fasting would make you feel better, fast. The good news is that science agrees with this wisdom. Researchers at Yale have done some preliminary work with rodents that implies that your body's appetite signals may just be in tune with what your body needs.[5] And since we should never forget that our bodies are trying to protect us at all times, it makes total sense to me that our bodies would send us just the right signals when we are sick!

GENERAL QUESTIONS

What is the best time of day for my eating window?

As I mentioned chapter 6, we don't have studies that compare different eating window times with all other factors being equal. Yes, there are some theories that an earlier window may have benefits, but I'm waiting to see conclusive studies. While we wait, here's what I think about this topic: the "best" eating window isn't the one that is theoretically "best" based on laboratory research or a handful of studies. The *best* eating window is the one that feels right to *you*. For me, that is an evening eating window. Why? It's pretty simple. When I open my eating window early in the day, I have a hard time closing it. For me, an early eating window turns into all-day eating. It's a lot easier for me personally to delay my eating window to later in the day. I also sleep better when my eating window is later in the day. You may be the exact opposite, though. Perhaps you feel better eating early in the day, and when you eat earlier in the day, you sail through the rest of the day with no hunger. Perhaps you sleep better when you eat earlier rather than closer to bedtime. Follow your body's lead and do what feels right to you.

Even if scientific research definitively proves one day that a specific eating window is superior physiologically, never forget that you are designing an intermittent fasting lifestyle that you can do long term. Personally, I know what feels good to me, and I know what does not feel good to me. That's the best evidence out there. Never forget that in many ways, we are all a study of one.

Is a shorter eating window always better for weight loss?

If weight loss came down to only calories in / calories out, then the answer to this question would probably be yes. In a shorter eating window, you would likely eat less food, and less food should always equal more weight loss, right?

Actually, no. If you remember the discussion about how our bodies adapt over time to low-calorie dieting, you know that we don't want to follow a long-term, overly restrictive plan. Even though intermittent fasting is protective in many ways, we still don't want to overly restrict, even with IF.

Also, our bodies react differently to stresses. While fasting is generally a "good" stress (just as exercise is generally a "good" stress), there comes a point where it can be too much for your body. The key is that this is a different point for every person.

There are people who follow 23:1 for months or years and lose weight and feel great. On the flip side, there are people who have bodies that find 23:1 to be overly restrictive and a negative stress. Some bodies react better to a longer window. Maybe your sweet spot is 16:8. Likely, it is somewhere in between the two extremes.

So, never forget—less isn't always more, particularly when it comes to choosing your ideal eating window. Tweak it till it's easy!

Does my eating window have to be at the same time / the same length every day?

Absolutely not! Feel free to adjust your eating window as necessary. Shift it around to accommodate a special event. Shorten it when you are busy. Lengthen it when you need to. If you have a shorter fast one day, you'll likely even it out with a longer fast the next day. Never forget that IF is a lifestyle that is flexible and adaptable.

What if I get hungry during the fast?

There's hunger, and there's *hunger.* Yes, even when you have been living the intermittent fasting lifestyle for years, you'll have waves of mild hunger throughout the day. That's normal, and it's not a sign that anything is wrong with you. The key is that the hunger passes quickly, and you can go about your day with no issues. Stay busy, drink a clean-fast-approved beverage, and be amazed when you forget all about it!

If you have a hunger that is different—you're nauseous and/or shaky, and you just can't keep going—consider that to be a signal from your body to go ahead and eat. Over time, you'll learn the difference between mild hunger that isn't an emergency and *time to eat now!* hunger. There's a distinct difference. If you are still in the FAST Start, however, expect to be hungrier as your body adjusts to fasting. If you need to drop back to a more gradual plan, that's okay.

How should I handle social situations that occur when my eating window is closed? On a related note, how should I handle pressure to eat when I don't want to eat?

This is such a great question, because there will come a time when you are invited to participate in an event that occurs during the time of the day that you usually spend fasting. Or you'll be offered food by someone while outside of your eating window. This can be difficult for new IFers and for experienced IFers alike, since food is more than just nourishment for our bodies. Sharing a meal with others is about *so* much more than the food that is served. In some cultures, food is love, and I get it; when I prepare a meal for my family, I take great pleasure in knowing that they enjoy the food I am serving.

When faced with this dilemma, you have several options.

First, you could unabashedly decide to throw open your window and eat at a different time from when you normally do. I don't recommend that you do this every time someone offers you food, of course, but if the occasion is special and the food is window-worthy, it is absolutely fine to open your window early or leave it open longer on that special occasion. I never hesitate to have a longer eating window or eat early if it's a holiday, a special celebration, or if the food is special.

Let's say that the food is *not* window-worthy or that you aren't willing to open your window at that time. Remember—*you* are in charge of what goes into your body, not someone else.

You may feel pressured to eat to please others, but please get that out of your mind entirely. If you had a life-threatening food allergy to pea-nuts, you wouldn't eat peanuts just because someone offered them to you, would you? This is exactly the same thing. Okay, maybe this isn't exactly the same because opening your window early isn't life-threatening, but never forget that you are choosing intermittent fasting because of your health, so it doesn't serve you well to eat food that doesn't help you meet your health goals just because it's there or your aunt might be offended that you aren't eating her famous cookies. This is also a great time to learn the power of *delay*. Get used to saying, "Those look great! I'm not hungry right now, but I'd love to take one and eat it later!" (This is a trick all teach-ers already know, because kids love to offer you food that they are holding in their sweet-yet-germy little hands, and you definitely aren't going to ever eat that food, but they don't have to know that.) Or you can cheerfully say, "I've decided to delay, so I don't have to deny! I will eat later!" And the best news of all is that it's true!

Another issue is that you may feel self-conscious if others are eating and you are not. If the food is not window-worthy, then you should ab-solutely have no qualms about turning it down. If you are at a restaurant with others and the food is not something you want to eat, you do not have to eat. If everyone is in the break room at work eating doughnuts, you don't have to have a doughnut just because everyone else is. It was free-ing when I realized that most people are more worried about themselves than they are worried about what you are doing. If you don't make a big deal about it, they won't, either. Sit with them and enjoy your clean-fast-approved beverage and don't be at all self-conscious. (Funny story: One time, I went out to lunch with a bunch of teachers and about half of us were fasting. We didn't realize it until the server came to take our order. Oops. We left her a great tip to make up for taking up space that could have been filled with paying customers, and we had a great visit with one another even though some of us ate and some of us did not.)

You may also feel like you are missing out, because everyone else is eating and you "can't." Get that word *can't* of your mind. It isn't that you *can't*; it's that you don't *choose* to eat right then. At my work, when I was a teacher, lunch was a social time for teachers to spend in the teacher workroom. While it may have been hard at first to sit with others who were eating while I was fasting, I found it really helped me to think about what everyone was eating. Most people had frozen microwave meals, sandwiches, or leftovers. I could think ahead to the amazing dinner I would have later, and I realized that none of those workroom lunch options were as appealing to me as getting through the rest of my workday in the fasted state (with no afternoon slump!) so I could go home and feast without fear.

So, when you are faced with one of these situations and you choose not to eat, what do you say? Here's what I do *not* want you to do. I don't want you to feel like you have to lie to someone about what you are doing to excuse why you are not eating. Don't tell them you ate a big breakfast or that you are fasting because you have to have medical tests done. (Yes, these are both suggestions I have seen other people give.) What's wrong with a little white lie? To me, lying to others about what you are doing implies that what you are doing is something to be ashamed of or to hide. We aren't ashamed of IF; we know it is the health plan with the side effect of weight loss. We know that it is good for our bodies. So, we don't have to tell lies to hide it from other people. Reread chapter 24 to see tips about this concept.

Is it better to track my fasting hours or to track my eating window?

This is such an interesting conversation to have with other intermittent fasters because there is no right answer to the question, yet it is one that people feel *very* strongly about.

Personally, I find that it is more useful to me to track my eating window length. I feel best when my eating window is somewhere between two to six hours in length, and when I have an eating window beyond six hours, I usually feel like I have eaten too much food. I don't stress if I want to open my eating window earlier one day, because I know that I'll likely have a longer fast the next day. This is how it looks for me in practice: Yesterday, I opened my window a few hours earlier than usual due to a family event that happened at lunchtime. Because I had closed my window at 9:00 p.m. the day before, I fasted for only fifteen hours before opening my window at noon at the family event. I kept my window open for about five hours, from 12:00 p.m. to 5:00 p.m., and then I closed it because I had eaten enough food for the day, and I was pleasantly satisfied. Today, I will probably open my window at 5:00 p.m., and I will likely keep it open for four hours or so and close it by 9:00 p.m. That means I will have a twenty-four-hour fast before opening my window today. Yesterday's fast of fifteen hours (shorter than my normal fast) was balanced out by today's fast of twenty-four hours (longer than my normal fast). If my eating window is typically five hours or less, my *average* fasting time is always going to be nineteen hours or more. (One other thing that it's important for me to note: I could have chosen to not eat lunch with the family yesterday, and that would have been okay, too. It's fine to sit with family members who are eating and visit with them while I sip a clean-fast-approved beverage. I don't eat just because everyone else is eating; I eat only if the food is appealing and window-worthy, and yesterday's meal absolutely was.)

On the flip side, you may be someone who is interested in maximizing the benefits found in the fasted state, so you may find it motivational to always reach sixteen hours fasted (or eighteen, or twenty, or whatever goal you choose) before opening your eating window. I know many intermittent fasters prefer to think of it that way.

As I said, neither way is superior; it's all about what feels right to *you*.

What if my fasting / eating window times don't add up to twenty-four?

When we talk about the fasting/eating approaches, we always write them so they add up to twenty-four—16:8, 19:5, 20:4, and so on. That's because there are twenty-four hours in a calendar day, of course.

Still, people sometimes get worried because their numbers don't always "add up" to twenty-four in practice. This concept can be downright confusing. (You're probably not surprised to hear me say that you should *not* stress about this at all.)

Let me explain how this might look in practice. Let's say that you stop eating after dinner on Tuesday and close your window at 8:00 p.m. The next day, you open your window at 4:00 p.m. and eat until 9:00 p.m. Let's do the math. You fasted from 8:00 p.m. on Tuesday until 4:00 p.m. on Wednesday, which was a twenty-hour fast. Then, you had a five-hour eating window. If you add twenty plus five, that equals TWENTY-FIVE HOURS. What?!!?!? Is this some sort of new math?

Deep breath. It's okay. Yes, there are twenty-four hours in a calendar day. But in almost all situations, we fast overnight (not you, shift workers, but you're a special case). That means that your fasting time spans through *two* calendar days. For that reason, the numbers won't always add up neatly to twenty-four. And that is no big deal. Remember: Fast. Feast. Repeat. Don't get caught up in the tiny details like this one.

Can I do a twenty-four-hour fast every day?

Sure, if you want to! But probably not in practice. Let me explain. If you fast for twenty-four hours, you'll then need to have an eating window of some duration. Let's say that you open your eating window at 6:00 p.m. Even if you are a *really* quick eater, you'll have an eating window. Let's say you eat until 6:15 (which I wouldn't recommend, because that doesn't sound very enjoyable or like a long-term lifestyle). If you close your window at 6:15 p.m. and then fast for twenty-four hours, you will need to open your window at 6:15 the next night. If you continue this pattern, you'll be eating at 6:30, then 6:45, then 7:00, and so on just to get in a twenty-four-hour fast. Pretty soon, you'll be waking up in the middle of the night to open your window. So, *can* you do a twenty-four-hour fast every day? Sure. Will you? Probably not.

If fasting is so healthy, why don't I just fast for days/weeks/months until I get to my goal weight?

Quick! Reread chapter 9! There *is* such a thing as too much fasting. Even though fasting has hormonal and metabolic benefits, over-fasting can downregulate your metabolism over time. That's the last thing you want!

Can I split up my day into TWO eating windows? Meaning, have breakfast from 8:00 a.m. to 9:00 a.m., close my window, fast until dinner, and then eat from 6:00 p.m. to 7:00 p.m.?

I am sorry to be the bearer of bad news, but the answer is no. With a schedule such as the one you are describing, you would not receive the full benefits we expect from the fasted state, as you are eating again just as your body starts to reach the fat-burning stage. Instead, compress all eating experiences within *one* eating window, and count the hours from the first bite of food for the day to the last bite of food for the day.

My window is closing, and I'm not hungry. Should I eat more food now so I won't be hungry later?

This is a real dilemma for many people, particularly new IFers. We look ahead to the hours and hours of fasting stretching before us and think we need to eat something *now* so we won't be hungry *later*. Remember what I have taught you about appetite correction, and that is that you should never eat more food than your body wants or needs. Don't eat for future hunger; eat for current hunger. If you are satisfied, don't eat more food just because you think you should.

I already closed my window for the day, but I am STARVING. What should I do?

This is a real "listen to your body" moment. If you are genuinely hungry, eat. Remember—there is no such thing as the fasting patrol that will show up at your door and confront you. Make sure you are actually hungry, however, and not just bored. One way to determine if it is real hunger or boredom is to set a timer for thirty minutes. Tell yourself you can have something at the end of the thirty minutes if you really are hungry. You may just find that it passes and you really weren't hungry after all. Don't reopen your window just because something sounds good or other people are eating.

Help! I accidentally tasted food / sipped a non-fast-compliant beverage during the fast. What do I do?

First, don't panic. This happens to many people, particularly when they are starting out. Does it break the fast? Of course. Eating is never fasting. That being said, it was likely not much. Your best bet is to continue as if it didn't happen (and try not to do it again). If, however, you become shaky or nauseous within an hour or so, you should go ahead and eat something. That's a sign that your blood glucose has dropped (in response to an insulin release) and you need to eat.

Can I / should I have a "cheat" day?

I recommend that you NEVER have a cheat day when living an intermittent fasting lifestyle. Nope. No cheat days are allowed whatsoever.

Before you get too upset with the thought that you can never have a day where you "live a little," let me explain.

Cheating implies that you are doing something wrong. People cheat on their taxes. Students cheat on a test. A spouse may cheat on a partner. All are taboo.

This is important—you can't cheat on intermittent fasting because it is a lifestyle.

You may have a day where you choose to set fasting aside for a special occasion. That is not cheating; it is a planned indulgence. *You* are in control at all times.

You will also have a day from time to time where your ghrelin seems to be in overdrive, and you eat more food than you intended, perhaps making you feel physically ill. That is also not a "cheat." It is a learning experience. You soon realize that you don't feel well when you overeat. I think these are important lessons, and they help us internalize the important concept that we feel so much better when we follow an intermittent fasting lifestyle and stop eating when we are satisfied rather than stuffed.

So, a *cheat day*? It doesn't exist. Words are important! Have a feast day if your body needs it. Enjoy your special occasion. Zero guilt . . . because there's zero cheating in an intermittent fasting lifestyle.

How do I explain what I am doing to my children?

Parents, particularly parents of girls, wonder how to explain fasting to their children. We all know that kids are impressionable, and we don't want to pass on any disordered eating behaviors to them. What's a parent to do?

Of course, we know that fasting is healthy and not at all disordered eating, but how do we communicate this to our kids? I have found that children understand one concept immediately: **Growing bodies have different nutritional needs than bodies that are already grown.**

I have never met a kid who didn't understand that.

When you are trying to grow a body, you need to feed it more frequently. (Think about babies, who have to eat around the clock. They are growing at the fastest rate of their lives, so they eat the most often.) On the other hand, when your body is fully grown, you don't need to feed it so often.

When you do eat, let your kids see you eat with freedom and gusto! They'll see that you have a healthy relationship with food and eating, which is precisely want we want them to learn from us.

When you feed a meal to your kids and your eating window isn't open yet, take the time to sit with them and spend time with them. Just because you aren't eating, that doesn't mean that you can't have quality time together!

CAN I HAVE ___ WHILE FASTING?

Will I still lose weight if I don't follow the recommendations for a clean fast?

Stern teacher glance from me: "And why do you ask?" This is a typical rebel question, by the way.

This is the most important concept to take away from this book. If you are not sure that the clean fast is important, my homework assignment for you is to go reread the clean fast chapters again and again until the rationale behind the recommendations sinks in. I promise that the clean fast is where the magic is found. Take the Clean Fast Challenge and you'll understand for yourself.

If you want to experience the hormonal and metabolic benefits of fasting, you have to actually fast clean. Can you lose weight without the clean fast? Of course you can. Haven't we all lost weight in the past, prior to IF? The key is that we didn't maintain the loss long term, or we did metabolic damage to our bodies, or both.

Yes. You absolutely *can* lose weight without the clean fast. Heck, you might even lose weight on the scale more quickly than with the clean fast, because you don't experience the amazing body recomposition that the clean fast gives us. But never forget our goal; we aren't looking for *quick* weight loss on the scale. We are looking for *permanent* fat loss, while maintaining and building lean muscle mass and avoiding metabolic slow-down. To see those benefits, fast clean.

I saw a video that said it's okay to have _____ while fasting, but you say it isn't okay. Why is there disagreement about what to have while fasting?

Let me tell you something about myself to illustrate this point. Back in the day, when I didn't understand how the body worked and I was enjoying stevia in my coffee while thinking I was fasting, I looked for any evidence I could find that would support my wish to have that delicious and sweet coffee treat during the fast. So, I understand where you are coming from. Really, I do. If you look for "evidence" that something is okay, you *will* find it somewhere. Thank goodness I read Dr. Jason Fung's book *The Obesity Code* in 2016, and I finally understood the role increased insulin plays in our bodies. Once I understood how CPIR from even zero-calorie sweet tastes factored into the equation, that was all it took. #SteviaYouAreDeadToMe. (Sometimes people think this means I am anti-stevia completely. If you want to use stevia during your eating window, go for it. Just keep it out of the fast. I have realized I don't like the taste of stevia any longer, so I avoid it always, but if I liked it, I would have it during my eating window.)

So, whenever faced with conflicting advice for what is safe to consume during the fast, let's think about it this way. Go back to chapter 4 and revisit the three goals of the clean fast. Do you want to risk raising your insulin levels? Do you want to risk preventing your body from accessing your stored fat for fuel? Do you want to risk stopping your body from increasing autophagy during the fast? No, no, and no.

My belief is that I always want to err on the side of caution. If I found five sources telling me to avoid something during the fast and five sources telling me it's fine, I would most likely choose to go with the "avoid" recommendation. That's because I don't want to waste precious fasting time by consuming something that is wasting my efforts.

I heard an expert say that coffee and tea break the fast, and we should stick to water only. What's up with that?

There was a podcast interview a few years ago where one fasting expert claimed that coffee and tea break the fast and people should stick to water only. That was like a stick of dynamite! People in the fasting world shared the heck out of that interview for weeks, and suddenly everyone was concerned that coffee and tea broke the fast.

Funny story—the *same expert* who was interviewed on that podcast did another interview not too long after that, and in it, he said, "When I stand in line [at my favorite coffee shops], then I see almost 95 percent of people will get that coffee, come back to the milk and cream station, and then pour a lot of sugar and cream and drink their coffee. That's why we tell people, 'No. Drinking coffee outside that window is not allowed, because we know 95 percent of people do this.' But if some people can control and have only black coffee, then at least this should be okay in the first half of the day." Ha! So, his recommendations to avoid coffee were mainly because he knew people didn't want to fast clean.

I have fully researched the topic, and if I felt that coffee or tea interfered with the clean fast, I would tell you. Since coffee and tea are linked to both increased autophagy and increased fat burning, I am confident with my recommendation to include them in the clean fast.[6] If you are still not convinced, it's fine to avoid coffee and tea and stick to water!

What should I do about my medications and supplements? Do they break the fast?

When it comes to taking prescribed medications, you absolutely should never make any changes to your schedule without talking to your doctor and/or pharmacist. Please ask whether intermittent fasting affects the recommended dosages or timings for your specific medications, as that could be an issue. Some medications shouldn't ever be taken on an empty stomach, and others may cause issues when taken in the fasted state (such as causing your blood pressure or blood glucose levels to drop to unsafe levels).

Notice that I didn't answer the question as to whether medications break the fast, and that's because it is actually irrelevant. If you *need* to take a medication, then it's important for you to take it, using your doctor's guidance for how intermittent fasting fits into the mix.

As for vitamins and supplements, there is no easy answer to this question. That's because every formulation is going to be different. When a supplement is clearly food-like (check the ingredients), it's best to keep it within your eating window. Many supplements and vitamins actually work better when you have them with food.

I have to take a daily medication with food, and the recommended dosage times fall within my fasting time. What should I do?

The very best person to have this conversation with is your health care provider or pharmacist. He or she will be knowledgeable about your specific medications, the timings, and what foods should or should not be consumed with them. You may be surprised to find that your doctor can adjust your medication or timing so that you don't have to take them during the fast. It doesn't hurt to ask!

If you absolutely have to take medications with food during your fast, the bad news is that food does break the fast. Being compliant with your medications is, however, much more important than keeping the fast. If you must take a medication with food and it's during your fasting time, choose something that will cause a smaller insulin response. Anything that is higher in fat and lower in protein and carbohydrates would be a better choice, as fat by itself is likely to cause a smaller insulin release than something composed of carbohydrates or protein. While it may sound weird, consider taking your medications with a little butter or cream cheese. If you have a medication that shouldn't be taken with dairy, try a couple of macadamia nuts or a small handful of leafy greens (while leafy greens are not high fat, they are the go-to recommendation by Dr. Jason Fung in his book *The Complete Guide to Fasting*, because they are low in calories and won't interrupt the fast as much as other options might).

How do I know if _____ is okay to have during the fast?

I get this question all the time. Fun fact: this question is usually about tea, because there are so many beverages called "tea" that aren't really tea.

Whenever you aren't sure if something is okay to have during the fast, whether it's tea or whether it's something else, go back to the diagram illustrating the clean fast. Look at the ingredients list and compare the ingredients against the Yes and No lists on the diagram. If it has only ingredients from the Yes column, it's fine. If it has ingredients from the No column, you know it doesn't work. And when in doubt, leave it out.

Teas are still going to be tricky, but use that same technique with teas. First, check the ingredients list for hidden added flavors, and if flavors are added, it's clearly a no. Also remember that you want to avoid any food-like flavors and stick with teas that have a bitter flavor profile.

Does Communion break the fast?

Technically, yes. When you partake in Communion, you are ingesting something that will "break the fast." However, Communion is a spiritual practice and a religious observance. For that reason, participate in Communion according to your religious traditions and don't give it another thought. Go about your day as if it didn't happen.

If you find that you become ravenous or shaky after participating, then please go ahead and open your eating window. It's also fine to shift your eating window on those days to accommodate the timing of Communion. Remember, *you* are in charge, and IF is a lifestyle. You must design an IF schedule that fits your life, and this is one example of that.

Does vaping / chewing tobacco / smoking break the fast?

Let's talk about vaping first. Vaping liquids frequently have fruity or candy-like flavors, which is part of their appeal. Since we already know that we want to avoid sweet or fruity flavors (or any food-like flavors) while fasting, it makes sense that you would not want to vape sweet or food-like liquids during the fast. If you do want to vape, choose a flavorless liquid.

Chewing tobaccos usually have flavorings and/or sweeteners added to them. Since we avoid flavorings and sweeteners during the fast, those would be a no for the clean fast.

To answer the question about smoking cigarettes during the fast, I went to the R. J. Reynolds Tobacco Company website. RJR is an American cigarette manufacturer in the same city where I went to college, Winston-Salem, North Carolina. Yes, the entire city has the same name as two types of cigarettes. (Fun fact: When I was doing my student teaching in 1989, we took our third-grade students on a field trip to the cigarette factory. Teachers received their very own packs of cigarettes at the end of the tour. The kids got candy. Good times.)

According to RJR's website, cigarettes may contain (among other things): apple juice concentrate, brown sugar, carob, chocolate liquor, cocoa, corn syrup, dextrose, fig extract, honey, invert sugar, molasses, pineapple juice concentrate, sucrose, sugar beet juice, and/or vanilla extract.[7] Those are only the food-like or sweet ingredients that I recognized from the long list of possible ingredients, but there were dozens of other ingredients.

I know that you are lighting the cigarette on fire and inhaling the smoke rather than ingesting the individual ingredients, but I have no idea how much of that sweetness message gets to the brain or whether it would initiate a cephalic phase insulin response. We do know that smoking is associated with both insulin resistance and an increased risk for type-2 diabetes, which could be a clue.[8,9]

The bottom line is, if you think of the fast as a time for healing and repair in the body and you want to make sure that you have a squeaky-clean fast, it would make sense that you wouldn't want to risk it by smoking, chewing tobacco, or vaping. If you currently use these products, I bet you have thought about quitting. Think of this as the perfect opportunity to do this positive thing for your health! You won't regret it. The good news is that a nicotine patch will *not* break the fast, and it can help you kick the habit.

Can I take exogenous ketones while fasting?

The answer to this is no. I explained the rationale behind this chapter 4, so go back to that chapter to read the full explanation. Save the money you would spend on these expensive supplements for the delicious foods you plan to eat in your eating window!

What can I have during the fast to combat bad breath?

Since gum and mints are completely out of the question, many fasters are at a loss when it comes to dealing with bad breath during the fast. I get it! I was a heavy gum-chewer back in the day; I purchased six-hundred-piece containers of my favorite gum and kept a supply with me at all times. Once I embraced the clean fast, however, I had to drop the gum habit.

Peppermint essential oil (food grade) is in the gray area, but many intermittent fasters use it successfully for breath freshening. Keep in mind that the gray area isn't a *yes*, it's a *maybe*. Make sure your body is fully adjusted to the clean fast before experimenting with gray area items, and if you feel shaky or ravenous after using, that is a sign it doesn't work for your body. Also, it's important to use essential oils safely. A tiny drop on your tongue is all it takes, and you should not be swallowing the oil. One technique that sounds weird but works well is to place a tiny drop on the back of your (clean) hand and lick it off. You can also add a few drops to water in a tiny spray bottle and spray it into your mouth as a homemade breath spray. (One thing to keep in mind— don't add peppermint oil to water and drink it like a water enhancer. We aren't trying to make our water more exciting. Keep the water you drink plain.)

Besides using peppermint oil, I find that simply swishing plain water around in my mouth or brushing my tongue with plain water helps a lot, particularly if I have coffee breath. I have also mastered the art of not breathing in someone's face, which is a great technique if all else fails.

Can I use flavored lip balm during the fast?

This may sound like a nutty question, but think about it—they actually do call them *flavors*. While I have never seen a study on lip balm and insulin release, it makes sense that there may be a small cephalic phase insulin response related to certain lip balm flavors. For that reason, it is likely safest to choose a lip balm that doesn't "taste" like a sweet treat. I use a peppermint-flavored lip balm with no problems, but I wouldn't pick an option that was fruity or "vanilla cupcake" flavor.

Can I take a fiber supplement during the fast?

One of our goals is to have a period of digestive rest during the fast. For that reason, you want to avoid things that might stimulate the digestive processes. Save your fiber supplement for your eating window. Even better—focus on getting your fiber from nutrient-dense foods!

FOOD CHOICES / NUTRITION

What is the best thing to eat when I open my eating window?

I know that you are used to diet plans that tell you exactly what to eat, so prepare to be amazed by my answer: I can't answer that question for you.

And what I mean is that I can't answer that question for *you*.

Because your body is different from mine, the foods that work well for me might not work well for you. I tend to open my window with a combination of fats and carbs, such as cheese and crackers, guacamole and chips, hummus and pretzels, and so on. Those foods work well for me. Perhaps you'll feel better opening your window with veggie sticks and dressing or an apple with peanut butter. Whatever foods are delicious, satisfying, and make *you* feel great—that is how you should open your window. That is what is "best" for *you*.

And you will figure this out over time by trial and error.

I can tell you that certain foods are likely to *not* work well for most people to have when opening their window: highly processed sugary foods, such as cookies or sweet lattes, are likely to be a problem for many people, because a large hit of processed/sugary foods will spike your blood glucose. As a result of the rapid intake of quickly absorbed glucose, your body will release insulin quickly, and then your blood sugar may crash. If you have ever experienced that, you know it isn't pleasant at all.

Also, I wouldn't recommend opening your window with alcohol on its own. When you drink alcohol on an empty stomach, it gets into your system much more quickly, which can be dangerous. So, make sure to eat food if you are going to be drinking alcohol. Trust me on this one. Not that I know from personal experience, of course.

Should I count calories / carbs / fat / and so on during my eating window just to be sure that I don't overeat?

No! And if you don't remember why, go back and read three chapters in the Feast section: "Bio-Individuality," "The End of the Calorie," and "Appetite Correction: What Exactly Is This Hormonal Voodoo?" It's important to trust that you can learn how to eat without external controls such as calorie or macro counting. Freedom!

How can I make sure to get in all my daily calories with a shorter eating window?

If you are living an intermittent fasting lifestyle with the hopes that you'll tap into your stored fat for fuel and lose some weight, think about this—you aren't trying to get calories *in*. You already *got them in*. Now, you're trying to get them back *out*.

Traditional thoughts on calorie counting have made us worried that we won't know if we are eating too much (or enough) unless we count every calorie, but as I explained in chapter 15, there are so many flaws to that type of thinking.

When you live an intermittent fasting lifestyle, remember that your body taps into your fat stores for fuel during the clean fast. You are fueled by fat during the fast, and your body understands that you're well fueled! Refer to chapter 1 for a more in-depth explanation.

Why am I bingeing as soon as I open my eating window?

If you're asking this question, you're probably in your first two months of IF. As I explained in previous chapters, overeating is common at first as your body adjusts to IF. Remember, until your body learns to tap into stored fat for fuel during the fast, your body is still searching for an energy source.

If you are a few months in and this is still happening, reread chapter 16 and consider applying some of the strategies I recommend there. If that doesn't help, I have heard great things about a book called *Brain over Binge,* so I recommend that you check it out.

Do I need to worry about not getting enough nutrients since I'm eating less food?

While we do have recommended daily allowances for specific nutrients, it's important to keep in mind that foods are incredibly complex combinations of nutrients and other compounds that we really don't even fully understand. Rather than focusing on individual nutrients on a daily basis, it's more important to focus on your overall *pattern* of eating.[10] Make sure you are eating a wide variety of nutritious foods from day to day, and you should be fine. I'm pretty sure that I get more nutrients *now,* as an IFer, than I used to when I was eating the Standard American Diet all day long. If you are concerned, you can always add a high-quality vitamin to your eating window.

MEDICAL QUESTIONS

I feel shaky/nauseous during the fast. What should I do?

If you ever feel shaky, nauseous, or unwell during the fast, please eat. These are signs that your blood glucose has dropped, and it's important to break your fast when you feel unwell. This might happen if you are new to IF and your body hasn't yet adjusted. Don't try to push yourself too hard at first, and it is fine to ease in. It also might happen if you inadvertently consume something that results in an insulin release in your body. Remember the role of insulin—its job is to help your cells take in glucose from your bloodstream. Therefore, when you have a sudden rise in insulin, your blood glucose goes down in response. This explains the blood sugar crash you experience. If this happens, think back to what you may have consumed. If it was something from the Maybe or No lists on the clean fast chart, then you know that it truly is a *no* for your body during the fast.

Can I do IF with a medical condition?

If you have a medical condition and you are concerned whether intermittent fasting is right for you, this is an important conversation to have with your doctor or medical practitioner. Intermittent fasting may be an excellent choice for you, but it might not be appropriate for your unique situation. Even though it is a healthy practice for many people, it's important to make sure it is right for *your* body.

Will IF heal my medical condition?

Intermittent fasting is great for many health conditions, but it may or may not help you with yours. Our bodies are so very complex, so there are no guarantees that intermittent fasting will have a positive effect on your specific medical condition. Always make sure your doctor or medical professional knows what you are doing, and follow all medical advice. Don't use intermittent fasting as a substitute for standard medical treatment.

Why do I have constipation/diarrhea now that I have started IF?

Some new IFers are surprised to find that they have unexpected changes in their pooping habits when they begin a new IF regimen. It helps to realize that these changes are, in fact, common, and most people find that they resolve over time as their bodies adjust to IF.

Feeling constipated? One reason may be related to water balance within your body. We know that we are using stored glycogen during the fast. Each gram of glycogen is stored along with three to four grams of water.[11] As our bodies release this excess water, we may become dehydrated, which can contribute to constipation.

Another cause of constipation is that when you are fasting, you tend to take in less food, which can slow down the action of your digestive system.

Eating, on the other hand, "wakes up" your digestive system, which can lead to diarrhea for some people, particularly at first. Diarrhea could also be caused by a disturbance within your gut microbiome as you experience changes related to fasting (the good news is that fasting promotes a healthy gut microbiome balance, so if your gastric distress is related to gut microbiome changes, chances are it will resolve soon).

If these poop problems don't resolve themselves on their own, you can try a magnesium supplement for constipation. Magnesium is a nutrient that many of us are deficient in, so taking a supplement can kill two birds with one stone. Also, make sure that you're getting plenty of fiber and remaining hydrated.

I have noticed that I am losing my hair. What's going on? Is this common?
I went through this very thing myself when I spent the summer of 2014 trying to follow a keto diet, and it was terrifying. I lost a ton of hair, and I was concerned that I would be bald! Fortunately, that didn't happen.

Hair loss happens for a multitude of reasons. Your body reacts to what it perceives to be a stressor by starting the hair-fall process. This is called *telogen effluvium*. You can ask Uncle Google if you want to read more about it.

This usually occurs two to three months after the event that triggered it. Yes, intermittent fasting (or *any* lifestyle change) can be perceived by the body as a stressor. If this is happening to you, think back two to three months and see if something else stressful was going on at that time. If not, IF is likely the culprit.

The bad news is that once the hair fall process starts (assuming it *is* telogen effluvium in your case), it has to run its course. The good news is that your hair doesn't all fall out. The better news is that it comes back.

My doctor has never heard of intermittent fasting / says intermittent fasting only works because you reduce calories / says that intermittent fasting will slow my metabolism, and so on. Why doesn't my doctor know the current research on IF, and what can I do?
Rest assured—many forward-thinking and innovative physicians follow intermittent fasting lifestyles themselves, and many prescribe intermittent fasting to their patients. If your doctor is unfamiliar with the practice, you have a few options. First, you can share resources with your doctor. Point them straight to the scientific studies, because that may be the most convincing for them as a trained scientist (you may want to choose from the ones that I shared with you here in the reference section of this book). Or you could bring in a book written by a physician (such as one written by Dr. Jason Fung, who is having great success using intermittent fasting in his practice with his patients). Once your doctor sees the vast amount of scientific literature that supports the practice of intermittent fasting,

he or she will likely become a believer! I have heard stories from other intermittent fasters who shared IF with their doctors, usually after a stellar health change or weight loss, and their doctors then go on to try IF for themselves and also to recommend it to other patients. Stunning patient success turns skeptical doctors into believers!

What if your doctor is still not receptive? The bottom line is this: It's important to have a medical team that you can think of as your partners in health-care decisions. While you should never actively disregard or ignore medical advice, it is absolutely fine to find a new doctor who shares your health-care philosophies.

Is IF helpful for someone with PCOS?

A recent study showed that fasting showed multiple benefits for women who suffer from PCOS, which is polycystic ovary syndrome.[12] Since PCOS is linked to hyperinsulinemia, it makes sense that fasting would be beneficial.[13] In addition to fasting, someone with PCOS may want to take other measures to lower insulin levels, and a lower-carb approach may also be beneficial.

EXERCISE

What is the best time of day to work out?

As I mentioned in chapter 21, the best time is the one that works with your schedule and fits into your day. That being said, there's a lot to support the benefits of working out in a fasted state. Reread that section of chapter 21 to remember why!

My trainer told me that I had to have protein immediately before/after/during my workout. Is that true? And I'm worried that I am not getting in enough protein during my eating window. Don't I need to eat a lot of protein to build muscle?

The short answer is that you do *not* need to take in protein immediately before/after/during your workout. Go back to chapter 21 and reread the discussion about protein timing and working out for a more thorough explanation.

If you are a bodybuilder, however, you may be more concerned with increased protein needs. In that case, I would find a trainer or expert who understands how intermittent fasting and bodybuilding work together.

Can I take a pre-workout/post-workout/BCAAs/other exercise supplements during the fast?

Think back to chapter 3 and recall that scientists discovered that our bodies ramp up natural production of carnitine and your body also recycles BCAAs during fasting. For that reason, you don't *need* to take them in a supplement, and definitely not during the fast! Keep in mind that most of the recommendations for these products come from someone who is trying to sell them to you by convincing you that you need them.

Also, taking them in supplement form would break the fast due to the protein/food-like ingredients found in these supplements. If your goal is lowered insulin levels and increased autophagy during the fast, you don't want to take in any of these supplements.

TRACKING YOUR PROGRESS

Will I lose _____ pounds in _____ days/weeks/months?

We have all heard the spectacular promises made by diet plans: "Lose twelve pounds in your first week!" or "Drop three sizes in your first month!" Intermittent fasting is not like that. As I mentioned in chapter 18, IF is in many ways the exact opposite of the diet plans you have tried before. With traditional diet plans, your best week of loss is usually week 1, and then progress slows dramatically over time. Eventually, you plateau, followed by regaining all the weight you lost. With IF, that's not what happens. You may even gain a little weight at first as your body adjusts to fasting. Then your body may need some time to adapt (and to heal) before you can efficiently tap into your fat stores for fuel. Once you have made it through the FAST Start phase, expect a slow and steady rate of loss, with an average of about a pound per week. As long as your weekly average is trending slowly downward over time, you are making progress.

So, will you lose _____ pounds by a certain deadline? Please don't count on that! And don't put pressure on yourself to meet numerical weight-loss goals that are tied to a date. Remember that IF is for life, and so you have plenty of time to get to your body's natural weight. You can't rush the process.

Why am I losing clothing sizes but no pounds on the scale?

Go back to chapter 18 and read the section about body recomposition! As you lose fat and build muscle, your body shrinks in size and you need smaller clothes, but your weight may not be changing on the scale. Always trust your changing size more than you trust the scale!

Why am I losing pounds on the scale, but my size isn't changing?

This is the opposite problem from the previous question, and we do see it from time to time: someone will report that they are down a great deal on the scale, but their measurements haven't budged and they aren't fitting into smaller clothes. Anecdotally, I have heard some people who have lost as much as ten or twenty pounds of scale weight but have seen no changes in their measurements or clothing sizes. How could this be possible?

Inside our bodies, we have fat stashed in all sorts of places. You may have heard of something called *visceral fat,* which is said to be the most unhealthy kind of fat. It's the fat your body stores in your abdominal cavity and therefore around your internal organs. High levels of visceral fat are linked to all sorts of negative medical conditions, such as insulin resistance, type 2 diabetes, heart disease, and more.

During fasting, your body taps into fat from various places, and we *hope* we are tapping into this unhealthy visceral fat. We also hope we are clearing out other undesirable fat, such as the fat from a fatty liver.

So, if you see the scale trending downward but your size hasn't changed yet, don't fret or worry that there is something wrong with you. Instead, imagine that your body is clearing out the unhealthiest fat of all, and smile.

It's been three weeks, and I think I am eating too much food in my eating window. Plus, I'm gaining weight. Does that mean IF doesn't work for me?

Hang in there, new faster! And please go back and reread the FAST Start section. Remember that I don't want you to weigh yourself until the end of the first twenty-eight days, and this is why.

During the adjustment phase, your body hasn't yet regulated your satiety and hunger hormones, and you probably aren't even tapping into your stored fat for fuel efficiently yet. So, of *course* you are hungry! And when you are hungry, your body sends you the message to eat more food. It is really hard to resist that message, in fact.

So, yes. You'll find that you just may eat more food than your body needs at first. And yes, you may even gain weight.

This is why the FAST Start phase is so important. You have to let your body and hormones adjust first.

Trust me, new IFer. It's not that IF won't work for you. It's just that you need more time.

Why does my weight go up and down from day to day? Does that mean I'm doing something wrong?

Welcome to the reality of weight fluctuations! This is why it is so important to weigh yourself daily and calculate your weekly average for comparison purposes (or use an app that does the trending for you). Daily fluctuations are rather meaningless, and you have to get comfortable with them or else you have to throw your scale in the trash, as I did, or at the very least let someone you love hide it.

Our weight can fluctuate by several pounds from day to day (and even throughout the course of one day). When you get on the scale and it is up four pounds overnight, you did NOT gain four pounds of fat in that short time. Conversely, when you get on the scale and it is down four pounds overnight, you also didn't lose four pounds of fat in that short time.

The two main culprits for quick scale increases/decreases are food/waste volume and water balance.

If you eat more food than normal (or eat out at a restaurant), your body will be full of the excess food you ate. That food adds weight to your body as it passes through your digestive system. It also causes your body to retain water, because extra water is needed to process the larger amount of food.

One time, I went out of town for a girls' weekend. This was right after I hit my initial goal weight, and so I was still weighing myself daily. On Friday, I recorded my weight before I left home. Then I ate, drank, and was merry for the next three days. On Monday, back at home, I got on my scale only to find I was up *nine* pounds since Friday.

Does this mean that intermittent fasting had ruined my body and a weekend "off plan" means I was rapidly regaining weight thanks to a lowered metabolic rate?

No.

We ate at restaurants the whole weekend, including one that is famous for causing water retention: a Japanese steakhouse. I ate a *lot* of food. My fingers were puffy, and I could tell my system was full of that excess food. (I was literally "full of it," as the saying goes.)

Did I get upset and decide that I needed to do something radical, like fast for days and days to make up for the "weight gain"?

Again, the answer is no.

I hopped back on my regular IF pattern, and the excess weight was "gone" by Thursday.

My story illustrates a rather large fluctuation that would probably cause panic for most people, but even a smaller fluctuation of a pound or two might stress you out. Don't let it!

Again, remember the advice from chapter 18—only the overall trend matters. I promise.

PHYSIOLOGY OF FASTING

Isn't breakfast the most important meal of the day (a.k.a. the often quoted "If you don't eat breakfast, your metabolism will shut down and you will gain weight" or "Eating breakfast is linked to being a healthy weight, and people who skip breakfast are more likely to be overweight")?

Before we answer this question with some science, let's examine the roots of the myth that "breakfast is the most important meal of the day" and that not eating breakfast will cause you to have metabolic slowdown for all the livelong day. Everyone has heard this, and most of us not only believed it, we tried to follow the advice. Did you know that the foundation for this advice came from studies funded by the breakfast cereal companies? It's true! Here's just one example. A 2000 study that concluded with the statement "people who eat cereal . . . for breakfast have significantly lower body mass indices than those who skip breakfast or who eat meats and eggs for breakfast. This analysis provides evidence that skipping breakfast is not an effective way to manage weight" has this wording RIGHT THERE ON THE FIRST PAGE: "**Funding for this study was provided by the Kellogg Company**."[14] Shocker! Isn't it a *huge* coincidence that in a study funded by Kellogg, not only did they find evidence that skipping breakfast is not effective but they also concluded that the best breakfast of all wasn't eggs and bacon but was cereal? Thanks, Kellogg!

Good news! We don't have to take our breakfast advice from Kellogg after all. In 2019, scientists from Australia performed a systematic review of the scientific literature related to the advice to eat breakfast.[15] They looked at all the available data and concluded that there's "no evidence to support the notion that breakfast consumption promotes weight loss or that skipping breakfast leads to weight gain." So, feel free to have your cereal any time of day that fits with your preferred eating schedule, since there is no scientific basis for the notion that it has to be first thing in the morning.

Can we really get into ketosis while doing intermittent fasting with no dietary changes?

This question is a real sticking point for many because a lot of people have the mistaken idea that the only way to get into ketosis is to follow a ketogenic diet, which is not true. Fasting is also ketogenic.[16] If you can't remember how this process works, go back to chapter 1 and reread that section.

Should I measure my ketones to make sure I am getting into ketosis? If not, how can I be sure that I am burning fat during the fast?

As I explained in chapter 1, I don't recommend measuring ketone levels. Go back and reread that section to see why!

Why do I have ketone breath about an hour or so AFTER I eat? I'm eating carbs; shouldn't that knock me out of ketosis?

Once you ramp up your fat-burning superpower, your body is metabolically flexible. You can turn fat into ketones during the fast, which fuels your brain. When you eat, your body switches fuel sources to use the energy from the food you just consumed, and you no longer need those ketones that your body made during the fast. They have to go somewhere! You may notice that you are breathing them out about an hour or so after eating your first meal. No, you are not already "back in ketosis." You are simply getting rid of the ketones your body made during the fast.

At what point during the fast will I experience autophagy? I have heard it takes twenty-four hours of fasting or more. Others say it happens around hour sixteen of the fast. What's actually true?

This is a question that haunts the intermittent fasting world, and it would be really nice if we had an autophagy meter we could look at and know immediately that our bodies are engaged in cellular cleanup and repair. Of course, we don't have that. We do know that increased autophagy is linked to the state of ketosis. Go back to chapter 2 and reread that section for a refresher so you understand that this is something that varies from person to person (and even day to day) with no easy numerical answer. (And if anyone gives you a definite answer as to the moment you will experience increased autophagy, you should understand that they are just guessing based on averages.)

Why do I get so tired after breaking my fast? I want to take a nap!

Picture a pride of lions after a kill—they all take a nap! Digestion takes a lot of energy, so it is normal to be tired after eating. (You can also recall how you feel after Thanksgiving dinner.) This feeling of needing a nap after eating is much more pronounced for new IFers, by the way. Usually, it gets better over time, although I have to admit that I prefer the way I feel in the fasted state when I need to be fully mentally alert and sharp. This is why I have an evening eating window.

Why am I so cold during the fast? Does that mean my metabolism is slowing down?

When we are digesting food, our bodies create a great deal of heat, which helps keep us feeling warm and toasty. Also, when you are fasting, your body increases blood flow to your fat stores to mobilize fat for fuel, and this results in less blood flow to your extremities.[17] Brrr! It's normal, so drink something warm and bundle up when necessary.

I get really hot after I eat. Why is that?

When you eat, your body ramps up the digestive processes, creating heat. My husband says that he can literally feel the heat radiating off me sometimes after dinner. (I have taken my temperature using a thermometer when I felt this sensation, and my temperature has been as high as the 99 range, which is fascinating.) I like to think of it as my metabolism firing up to burn off my dinner.

I've read that if I follow IF long term, my body can adjust to my eating window and slow my metabolic rate. Is that true?

A slowed metabolism is one of the big concerns that those unfamiliar with IF often bring up. While it's true that our metabolic rate can slow if we over-restrict long term, when you follow a flexible intermittent fasting lifestyle and learn to listen to your body's hunger and satiety signals, you don't need to worry so much about metabolic adaptation. Reread chapter 1!

If you are concerned with your overall metabolic rate, watch your body temperature over time, which is a pretty good indicator of metabolic health. If your body temperature goes up, that's a good sign. If it goes down over time, that's a bad sign.[18]

If you find your body temperature is going down over time, I recommend incorporating ADF for a while, as described in chapter 7. That's a great option for giving your body the metabolic boost it may be looking for, thanks to the up days. Remember that the daily-eating-window approach isn't the only way to IF!

Personally, I have used the daily-eating-window approach for years now and have no problems with my metabolism that I can detect. I'm my own study of one, of course.

Help! I can't sleep. What can I do?

We do hear this from time to time, particularly from new IFers. Personally, I find that not eating enough during my eating window absolutely does affect my sleep quality.

Over time, experiment with different eating windows and foods to see what works better for you. As an example, I sleep better when I eat sufficient carbs and have an evening eating window, but I do *not* sleep well if I eat too much sugar or have too much wine. Someone else may find that they sleep better if they have a morning eating window.

Why does my blood sugar go up during the fast?

Please remember that I am not a doctor and that I am not giving you medical advice here. However, think back to chapter 1. When you are fasting, your liver releases stored glycogen to provide fuel for your brain and body. You can see this reflected in higher blood sugar levels; the blood glucose is coming from your body's own storage! Always follow your doctor's advice related to controlling your blood glucose, of course.

Why is my cholesterol higher now than before I started IF?

Again, please remember that I am not a medical doctor, so it's essential for you to follow the advice of your own medical practitioner. That being said, it's a well-known phenomenon that fat loss itself causes a temporary rise in blood cholesterol levels due to the release of stored fat. It's known as *transient hypercholesterolemia*.[19] *Transient* means *temporary*. Still, I would discuss this concept with your physician.

RECOMMENDED READING

Every teacher I know has stacks and stacks of books lying around, and I am no different. We also love to recommend our favorite books to others. In this section, I'm going to share just a few of my favorite books (and one spectacular research article) that relate to the topics here in *Fast. Feast. Repeat.* While I could have listed dozens of excellent books, I pared the list down to include only the essentials. Consider this your extra-credit assignment!

FAST

"Flipping the Metabolic Switch: Understanding and Applying Health Benefits of Fasting," Stephen D. Anton, Keelin Moehl, William T. Donahoo, Krisztina Marosi, Stephanie Lee, Arch G. Mainous III, Christiaan Leeuwenburgh, and Mark P. Mattson.

This is a journal article that was published in the February 2018 edition of *Obesity.* The entire text is available online for free, so search using the title or go to https://www.ncbi.nlm.nih.gov/pmc/articles/PMC5783752/. This article is an absolute treasure trove of the science behind fasting. It's pretty science-y, but after reading *Fast. Feast. Repeat.* I think you're ready for it!

The Obesity Code by Jason Fung and
The Diabetes Code by Jason Fung

After reading *Fast. Feast. Repeat.*, you may be ready for a deeper dive into the science explaining the connection between hormones and obesity. Start with *The Obesity Code* for the basics, but if you or anyone you love has been diagnosed with type 2 diabetes or is prediabetic, *The Diabetes Code* is a must-read.

FEAST

In Defense of Food by Michael Pollan

I am a huge Michael Pollan fan, and his television series *Cooked* inspired me to begin baking bread at home. One day, I would love to break bread with him. His book *In Defense of Food* will help you get rid of your own diet brain forever and embrace cooking and eating delicious *real* food. After reading this book, you will understand that food is supposed to be a pleasure and not a source of angst, and you will understand why we are all so confused to begin with.

The Diet Myth by Tim Spector

My copy of this book has highlights everywhere and twenty-seven ratty sticky-note tabs hanging off it, so you can see I have read and reread this excellent book over the years. Tim Spector is a gut researcher who also studies twins, teasing out what makes us unique. Is it our genes? Our gut microbiomes? Or an interplay between the two? In this book, Spector shares his fascinating work in a way that is easy to read and keeps you turning the pages like you're reading a thriller.

AC: The Power of Appetite Correction by Bert Herring

This little book changed my life in so many ways because it taught me that I didn't need to count calories ever again. Learning to trust my body's appestat was life-changing. I trust my body when it tells me I have had enough, and I also trust my body when it tells me that I need to eat more food. Thank you, Dr. Herring, for putting this concept into such a small but powerful phrase! Understanding appetite correction will set you free, just as it did me.

REPEAT

Mindset by Carol Dweck

Carol Dweck is a psychologist with decades of research into the science behind achievement and success. This book changed my life in so many ways because it so clearly explains the importance of cultivating the right mind-set in ourselves, our kids, and anyone we hope to inspire (employees, coworkers, and family members). When you apply the principles Dweck shares, you not only change yourself, you can also use the tools in your interactions with all the important people in your life.

You Are the Placebo by Joe Dispenza

I tried to figure out how to explain this book in my own words, but really, the description on the back cover says it best: "*You Are the Placebo* combines the latest research in neuroscience, biology, hypnosis, behavioral conditioning, and quantum physics to demystify the workings of the placebo effect . . . and show how the seemingly impossible can become possible." Yep. That's what the book is about! Read this one with an open mind and get ready to be amazed.

NOTES

Do you love science as much as I do, or do you still have questions about some of the concepts in this book? Rather than take my word for it (or whenever you want to know more), I want you to go straight to these original sources and dig into the information for yourself. My goal throughout this book has been to accurately represent the scientific research that I presented to you within these pages.

INTRODUCTION: THE DISMAL TRUTH ABOUT DIETS

1. Lowe MR, Doshi SD, Katterman SN, Feig EH. Dieting and restrained eating as prospective predictors of weight gain. *Front Psychol.* 2013;4:577. doi:10.3389/fpsyg.2013.00577
2. Kalm LM, Semba RD. They starved so that others be better fed: Remembering Ancel Keys and the Minnesota Experiment. *J Nutr.* 2005;135(6):1347–1352. doi:10.1093/jn/135.6.1347
3. Fothergill E, Guo J, Howard L, et al. Persistent metabolic adaptation 6 years after "The Biggest Loser" competition. *Obesity (Silver Spring).* 2016;24(8):1612–1619. doi:10.1002/oby.21538
4. Rosenbaum M, Hirsch J, Gallagher DA, Leibel RL. Long-term persistence of adaptive thermogenesis in subjects who have maintained a reduced body weight. *Am J Clin Nutr.* 2008;88(4):906–912. doi:10.1093/ajcn/88.4.906
5. Melby CL, Paris HL, Foright RM, Peth J. Attenuating the biologic drive for weight regain following weight loss: Must what goes down always go back up? *Nutrients.* 2017;9(5). doi:10.3390/nu9050468
6. Tremblay A, Royer M-M, Chaput J-P, Doucet É. Adaptive thermogenesis can make a difference in the ability of obese individuals to lose body weight. *Int J Obes.* 2013;37:759–764. doi:10.1038/ijo.2012.124

1: IGNITE YOUR FAT-BURNING SUPERPOWER

1. Crofts CAP. Hyperinsulinemia: A unifying theory of chronic disease? *Diabesity.* 2015;1(4):34. doi:10.15562/diabesity.2015.19

2. Duncan RE, Ahmadian M, Jaworski K, Sarkadi-Nagy E, Sul HS. Regulation of lipolysis in adipocytes. *Annu Rev Nutr.* 2007;27:79–101. doi:10.1146/annurev.nutr.27.061406.093734

3. Webber J, Macdonald IA. The cardiovascular, metabolic and hormonal changes accompanying acute starvation in men and women. *Br J Nutr.* 1994;71(3):437–447.

4. Polonsky KS, Given BD, Van Cauter E. Twenty-Four-Hour Profiles and Pulsatile Patterns of Insulin Secretion in Normal and Obese Subjects.

5. Müller MJ, Enderle J, Bosy-Westphal A. Changes in energy expenditure with weight gain and weight loss in humans. *Curr Obes Rep.* 2016;5(4):413–423. doi:10.1007/s13679-016-0237-4

6. Webber, Macdonald. The cardiovascular, metabolic and hormonal changes.

7. Mansell PI, Fellows IW, Macdonald IA. Enhanced thermogenic response to epinephrine after 48-h starvation in humans. *Am J Physiol Integr Comp Physiol.* 1990;258(1):R87–R93. doi:10.1152/ajpregu.1990.258.1.R87

8. Anton SD, Moehl K, Donahoo WT, et al. Flipping the metabolic switch: Understanding and applying the health benefits of fasting. *Obesity (Silver Spring).* 2018;26(2):254–268. doi:10.1002/oby.22065

9. Mattson MP, Longo VD, Harvie M. Impact of intermittent fasting on health and disease processes. *Ageing Res Rev.* 2017;39:46–58. doi:10.1016/j.arr.2016.10.005

10. Ruderman N, Meyers M, Chipkin S, Tornheim K. Hormone-Fuel Interrelationships: Fed State, Starvation, and Diabetes Mellitus | Oncohema Key. https://oncohemakey.com/hormone-fuel-interrelationships-fed-state-starvation-and-diabetes-mellitus/. Accessed August 6, 2019.

11. Smith RL, Soeters MR, Wüst RCI, Houtkooper RH. Metabolic flexibility as an adaptation to energy resources and requirements in health and disease. *Endocr Rev.* 2018;39(4):489–517. doi:10.1210/er.2017-00211

12. Ibid.

13. McPherron AC, Guo T, Bond ND, Gavrilova O. Increasing muscle mass to improve metabolism. *Adipocyte.* 2013;2(2):92–98. doi:10.4161/adip.22500

14. Varady KA. Intermittent versus daily calorie restriction: Which diet regimen is more effective for weight loss? *Obes Rev.* 2011;12(7):e593–e601. doi:10.1111/j.1467-789X.2011.00873.x

15. Salgin B, Marcovecchio ML, Hill N, Dunger DB, Frystyk J. The effect of prolonged fasting on levels of growth hormone–binding protein and free growth hormone. *Growth Horm IGF Res.* 2012;22(2):76–81. doi:10.1016/j.ghir.2012.02.003

16. Ho KY, Veldhuis JD, Johnson ML, et al. Fasting enhances growth hormone secretion and amplifies the complex rhythms of growth hormone secretion in man. *J Clin Invest.* 1988;81(4):968–975. doi:10.1172/JCI113450

17. Monson JP, Drake WM, Carroll PV, Weaver JU, Rodriguez-Arnao J, Savage MO. Influence of growth hormone on accretion of bone mass. *Horm Res Paediatr.* 2002;58(1):52–56. doi:10.1159/000064765

18. Bex M, Bouillon R. Growth hormone and bone health. *Horm Res Paediatr.* 2003;60(3):80–86. doi:10.1159/000074507

19. Dioufa N, Schally AV, Chatzistamou I, et al. Acceleration of wound healing by growth hormone-releasing hormone and its agonists. *Proc Natl Acad Sci USA.* 2010;107(43):18611. doi:10.1073/PNAS.1013942107

20. Lal SO, Wolf SE, Herndon DN. Growth hormone, burns and tissue healing. *Growth Horm IGF Res.* 2000;10:S39–S43. doi:10.1016/S1096-6374(00)80008-8

2: INTERMITTENT FASTING:
THE HEALTH PLAN WITH A SIDE EFFECT OF WEIGHT LOSS

1. Perlman RL. Mouse models of human disease: An evolutionary perspective. *Evol Med Public Heal.* 2016;2016(1):170–176. doi:10.1093/emph/eow014

2. Crofts CAP. Hyperinsulinemia: A unifying theory of chronic disease? *Diabesity.* 2015;1(4):34. doi:10.15562/diabesity.2015.19

3. Webber J, Macdonald IA. The cardiovascular, metabolic and hormonal changes accompanying acute starvation in men and women. *Br J Nutr.* 1994;71(3):437–447.

4. Sutton EF, Beyl R, Early KS, Cefalu WT, Ravussin E, Peterson CM. Early time-restricted feeding improves insulin sensitivity, blood pressure, and oxidative stress even without weight loss in men with prediabetes. *Cell Metab.* 2018;27. doi:10.1016/j.cmet.2018.04.010

5. Gabel K, Kroeger CM, Trepanowski JF, et al. Differential effects of alternate-day fasting versus daily calorie restriction on insulin resistance. *Obesity.* July 2019:oby.22564. doi:10.1002/oby.22564

6. Mattson MP, Longo VD, Harvie M. Impact of intermittent fasting on health and disease processes. *Ageing Res Rev.* 2017;39:46–58. doi:10.1016/j.arr.2016.10.005

7. Anton SD, Moehl K, Donahoo WT, et al. Flipping the metabolic switch: Understanding and applying the health benefits of fasting. *Obesity (Silver Spring).* 2018;26(2):254–268. doi:10.1002/oby.22065

8. Patterson RE, Sears DD. Metabolic effects of intermittent fasting. *Annu Rev Nutr.* 2017;37(1):371–393. doi:10.1146/annurev-nutr-071816-064634

9. Dinicolantonio JJ, Mccarty M. Autophagy-induced degradation of Notch1, achieved through intermittent fasting, may promote beta cell neogenesis: Implications for reversal of type 2 diabetes. *Open Heart.* 2019;6:1028. doi:10.1136/openhrt-2019-001028

10. Furmli S, Elmasry R, Ramos M, Fung J. Therapeutic use of intermittent fasting for people with type 2 diabetes as an alternative to insulin. *BMJ Case Rep.* 2018;2018. doi:10.1136/bcr-2017-221854

11. Hutchison AT, Regmi P, Manoogian ENC, et al. Time-restricted feeding improves glucose tolerance in men at risk for type 2 diabetes: A randomized crossover trial. *Obesity.* 2019;27(5):oby.22449. doi:10.1002/oby.22449

12. Horne BD, Muhlestein JB, May HT, et al. Relation of routine, periodic fasting to risk of diabetes mellitus, and coronary artery disease in patients undergoing coronary angiography. *Am J Cardiol.* 2012;109(11):1558–1562. doi:10.1016/j.amjcard.2012.01.379

13. Dinicolantonio, Mccarty. Autophagy-induced degradation of Notch1.

14. Risk Factors: Chronic Inflammation - National Cancer Institute. https://www.cancer.gov/about-cancer/causes-prevention/risk/chronic-inflammation. Accessed July 5, 2019.

15. Anton, Moehl, Donahoo, et al. Flipping the metabolic switch.

16. Mattson, Longo, Harvie. Impact of intermittent fasting.

17. Sutton, Beyl, Early, Cefalu, Ravussin, Peterson. Early time-restricted feeding improves insulin sensitivity.

18. Youm Y-H, Nguyen KY, Grant RW, et al. The ketone metabolite β-hydroxybutyrate blocks NLRP3 inflammasome–mediated inflammatory disease. *Nat Med.* 2015;21(3):263–269. doi:10.1038/nm.3804

19. Aksungar FB, Topkaya AE, Akyildiz M. Interleukin-6, C-reactive protein and biochemical parameters during prolonged intermittent fasting. *Ann Nutr Metab.* 2007;51(1):88–95. doi:10.1159/000100954

20. Faris MA, Kacimi S, Al-Kurd RA, et al. Intermittent fasting during Ramadan attenuates proinflammatory cytokines and immune cells in healthy subjects. *Nutr Res.* 2012;32(12):947–955. doi:10.1016/J.NUTRES.2012.06.021

21. Johnson JB, Summer W, Cutler RG, et al. Alternate day calorie restriction improves clinical findings and reduces markers of oxidative stress and inflammation in overweight adults with moderate asthma. *Free Radic Biol Med.* 2007;42(5):665–674. doi:10.1016/j.freeradbiomed.2006.12.005

22. Hayter SM, Cook MC. Updated assessment of the prevalence, spectrum and case definition of autoimmune disease. *Autoimmun Rev.* 2012;11(10):754–765. doi:10.1016/J.AUTREV.2012.02.001

23. Liu Y, Yu Y, Matarese G, La Cava A. Fasting-induced hypoleptinemia expands functional regulatory T cells in systemic lupus erythematosus. *J Immunol.* 2012;188(5):2070–2073. doi:10.4049/jimmunol.1102835

24. Regulation of Inflammation in Autoimmune Diseases. https://www.hindawi.com/journals/jir/si/495348/cfp/. Accessed July 6, 2019.

25. Sköldstam L, Larsson L, Lindström FD. Effect of fasting and lactovegetarian diet on rheumatoid arthritis. *Scand J Rheumatol.* 1979;8(4):249–255.

26. Said MSM, Vin SX, Azhar NA, et al. The effects of the Ramadan month of fasting on disease activity in patients with rheumatoid arthritis. *Turkish J Rheumatol.* 2013;28(3):189–194. doi:10.5606/tjr.2013.3147

27. Damiani G, Watad A, Bridgewood C, et al. The impact of Ramadan fasting on the reduction of PASI score, in moderate-to-severe psoriatic patients: A real-life multicenter study. *Nutrients.* 2019;11(2). doi:10.3390/nu11020277

28. Choi IY, Piccio L, Childress P, et al. A diet mimicking fasting promotes regeneration and reduces autoimmunity and multiple sclerosis symptoms. *Cell Rep.* 2016;15(10):2136–2146. doi:10.1016/j.celrep.2016.05.009

29. Mattson, Longo, Harvie. Impact of intermittent fasting.

30. Anton, Moehl, Donahoo, et al. Flipping the metabolic switch.

31. Varady KA, Bhutani S, Church EC, Klempel MC. Short-term modified alternate-day fasting: A novel dietary strategy for weight loss and cardioprotection in obese adults. *Am J Clin Nutr.* 2009;90(5):1138–1143. doi:10.3945/ajcn.2009.28380

32. Horne BD, May HT, Anderson JL, et al. Usefulness of routine periodic fasting to lower risk of coronary artery disease among patients undergoing coronary angiography. *Am J Cardiol.* 2008;102(7):814–819. doi:10.1016/j.amjcard.2008.05.021

33. Sutton, Beyl, Early, Cefalu, Ravussin, Peterson. Early time-restricted feeding improves insulin sensitivity.

34. Aksungar, Topkaya, Akyildiz. Interleukin-6, C-reactive protein.

35. Wan R, Ahmet I, Brown M, et al. Cardioprotective effect of intermittent fasting is associated with an elevation of adiponectin levels in rats. *J Nutr Biochem.* 2010;21(5):413–417. doi:10.1016/j.jnutbio.2009.01.020

36. Anton, Moehl, Donahoo, et al. Flipping the metabolic switch.

37. Mattson, Longo, Harvie. Impact of intermittent fasting.

38. Lee J, Seroogy KB, Mattson MP. Dietary restriction enhances neurotrophin expression and neurogenesis in the hippocampus of adult mice. *J Neurochem.* 2002;80(3):539–547. doi:10.1046/j.0022-3042.2001.00747.x

39. Mattson MP. Energy intake, meal frequency, and health: A neurobiological perspective. *Annu Rev Nutr.* 2005;25(1):237–260. doi:10.1146/annurev.nutr.25.050304.092526

40. Anton, Moehl, Donahoo, et al. Flipping the metabolic switch.

41. Li L, Wang Z, Zuo Z. Chronic intermittent fasting improves cognitive functions and brain structures in mice. Xie Z, ed. *PLOS ONE.* 2013;8(6):e66069. doi:10.1371/journal.pone.0066069

42. Halagappa VKM, Guo Z, Pearson M, et al. Intermittent fasting and caloric restriction ameliorate age-related behavioral deficits in the triple-transgenic mouse model of Alzheimer's disease. *Neurobiol Dis.* 2007;26(1):212–220. doi:10.1016/J.NBD.2006.12.019

43. Mattson, Longo, Harvie. Impact of intermittent fasting.

44. Mattson. Energy intake, meal frequency, and health.

45. Hussin NM, Shahar S, Teng NIMF, Ngah WZW, Das SK. Efficacy of fasting and calorie restriction (FCR) on mood and depression among ageing men. *J Nutr Health Aging.* 2013;17(8):674–680. doi:10.1007/s12603-013-0344-9

46. Ding H, Zheng S, Garcia-Ruiz D, et al. Fasting induces a subcutaneous-to-visceral fat switch mediated by microRNA-149-3p and suppression of PRDM16. *Nat Commun.* 2016;7(1):11533. doi:10.1038/ncomms11533

47. Anton, Moehl, Donahoo, et al. Flipping the metabolic switch.

48. Ding, Zheng, Garcia-Ruiz, et al. Fasting induces a subcutaneous-to-visceral fat switch.

49. Anton, Moehl, Donahoo, et al. Flipping the metabolic switch.

50. Mattson, Longo, Harvie. Impact of intermittent fasting.
51. Arnold JW, Roach J, Azcarate-Peril MA. Emerging technologies for gut microbiome research. *Trends Microbiol.* 2016;24(11):887–901. doi:10.1016/j. tim.2016.06.008
52. Malla MA, Dubey A, Kumar A, Yadav S, Hashem A, Abd Allah EF. Exploring the human microbiome: The potential future role of next-generation sequencing in disease diagnosis and treatment. *Front Immunol.* 2018;9:2868. doi:10.3389/fimmu.2018.02868
53. Castaner O, Goday A, Park Y-M, et al. The gut microbiome profile in obesity: A systematic review. *Int J Endocrinol.* 2018;2018:4095789. doi:10.1155/2018/4095789
54. Alang N, Kelly CR. Weight gain after fecal microbiota transplantation. *Open Forum Infect Dis.* 2015;2(1):ofv004. doi:10.1093/ofid/ofv004
55. Patterson, Sears. Metabolic effects of intermittent fasting.
56. Lee C, Raffaghello L, Brandhorst S, et al. Fasting cycles retard growth of tumors and sensitize a range of cancer cell types to chemotherapy. *Sci Transl Med.* 2012;4(124):124ra27. doi:10.1126/scitranslmed.3003293
57. Harvie MN, Howell T. Could intermittent energy restriction and intermittent fasting reduce rates of cancer in obese, overweight, and normal-weight subjects? A summary of evidence. *Adv Nutr.* 2016;7(4):690–705. doi:10.3945/an.115.011767
58. Rabin-Court A, Rodrigues MR, Zhang X-M, Perry RJ. Obesity-associated, but not obesity-independent, tumors respond to insulin by increasing mitochondrial glucose oxidation. Tan M, ed. *PLOS ONE.* 2019;14(6):e0218126. doi:10.1371/journal.pone.0218126
59. Harvie, Howell. Could intermittent energy restriction and intermittent fasting.
60. Lee, Raffaghello, Brandhorst, et al. Fasting cycles retard growth.
61. Mattson, Longo, Harvie. Impact of intermittent fasting.
62. Descamps O, Riondel J, Ducros V, Roussel A-M. Mitochondrial production of reactive oxygen species and incidence of age-associated lymphoma in OF1 mice: Effect of alternate-day fasting. *Mech Ageing Dev.* 2005;126(11):1185–1191. doi:10.1016/J.MAD.2005.06.007
63. Kirkin V. History of the selective autophagy research: How did it begin and where does it stand today? *J Mol Biol.* May 2019. doi:10.1016/J.JMB.2019.05.010
64. Upcycling. https://en.wikipedia.org/wiki/Upcycling. Accessed July 6, 2019.
65. Rabinowitz JD, White E. Autophagy and metabolism. *Science.* 2010;330(6009):1344–1348. doi:10.1126/science.1193497
66. Fung J. How Much Protein Is Excessive? Intensive Dietary Management (IDM). https://idmprogram.com/how-much-protein-is-excessive/. Accessed July 6, 2019.
67. Dunlop EA, Tee AR. mTOR and autophagy: A dynamic relationship governed by nutrients and energy. *Semin Cell Dev Biol.* 2014;36:121–129. doi:10.1016/J. SEMCDB.2014.08.006
68. Rabinowitz, White. Autophagy and metabolism.

69. Takagi A, Kume S, Maegawa H, Uzu T. Emerging role of mammalian autophagy in ketogenesis to overcome starvation. *Autophagy.* 2016;12(4):709–710. doi:10.1080/15548627.2016.1151597

70. McCarty MF, DiNicolantonio JJ, O'Keefe JH. Ketosis may promote brain macroautophagy by activating Sirt1 and hypoxia-inducible factor-1. *Med Hypotheses.* 2015;85(5):631–639. doi:10.1016/J.MEHY.2015.08.002

71. Mizushima N, Yamamoto A, Matsui M, Yoshimori T, Ohsumi Y. In vivo analysis of autophagy in response to nutrient starvation using transgenic mice expressing a fluorescent autophagosome marker. *Mol Biol Cell.* 2004;15(3):1101. doi: 10.1091/MBC.E03-09-0704

72. Ibid.

3: FASTING: THE REAL-LIFE FOUNTAIN OF YOUTH?

1. Teruya T, Chaleckis R, Takada J, Yanagida M, Kondoh H. Diverse metabolic reactions activated during 58-hr fasting are revealed by non-targeted metabolomic analysis of human blood. *Sci Rep.* 2019;9(1):854. doi:10.1038/s41598-018-36674-9

2. Canani RB, Costanzo M Di, Leone L, Pedata M, Meli R, Calignano A. Potential beneficial effects of butyrate in intestinal and extraintestinal diseases. *World J Gastroenterol.* 2011;17(12):1519–1528. doi:10.3748/wjg.v17.i12.1519

3. Lee J, Giordano S, Zhang J. Autophagy, mitochondria and oxidative stress: Cross-talk and redox signalling. *Biochem J.* 2012;441(2):523–540. doi:10.1042/BJ20111451

4. Wang C, Youle RJ. The role of mitochondria in apoptosis. *Annu Rev Genet.* 2009;43:95–118. doi:10.1146/annurev-genet-102108-134850

5. Kaur J, Debnath J. Autophagy at the crossroads of catabolism and anabolism. *Nat Rev Mol Cell Biol.* 2015;16(8):461–472. doi:10.1038/nrm4024

6. Ibid.

7. Feldscher K. Intermittent Fasting May Be Center Of Increasing Lifespan—Harvard Gazette. *Harvard Gazette.* https://news.harvard.edu/gazette/story/2017/11/intermittent-fasting-may-be-center-of-increasing-lifespan/. Accessed July 5, 2019.

8. Han Y-M, Bedarida T, Ding Y, et al. β-hydroxybutyrate prevents vascular senescence through hnRNP A1-mediated upregulation of Oct4. *Mol Cell.* 2018;71(6):1064–1078.e5. doi:10.1016/j.molcel.2018.07.036

9. Mihaylova MM, Cheng C-W, Cao AQ, et al. Fasting activates fatty acid oxidation to enhance intestinal stem cell function during homeostasis and aging. *Cell Stem Cell.* 2018;22(5):769–778.e4. doi:10.1016/j.stem.2018.04.001

10. Anton SD, Moehl K, Donahoo WT, et al. Flipping the metabolic switch: Understanding and applying the health benefits of fasting. *Obesity (Silver Spring).* 2018;26(2):254–268. doi:10.1002/oby.22065

11. Mitchell SJ, Bernier M, Mattison JA, et al. Daily fasting improves health and survival in male mice independent of diet composition and calories. *Cell Metab.* 2019;29(1):221–228.e3. doi:10.1016/j.cmet.2018.08.011

4: THE MAGIC IS IN THE CLEAN FAST!
LEARN WHY WE FAST CLEAN

1. Satoh-Kuriwada S, Shoji N, Miyake H, Watanabe C, Sasano T. Effects and mechanisms of tastants on the gustatory-salivary reflex in human minor salivary glands. *Biomed Res Int.* 2018;2018:1–12. doi:10.1155/2018/3847075
2. Tonosaki K, Hori Y, Shimizu Y, Tonosaki K. Relationships between insulin release and taste. *Biomed Res.* 2007;28(2):79–83.
3. Just T, Pau HW, Engel U, Hummel T. Cephalic phase insulin release in healthy humans after taste stimulation? *Appetite.* 2008;51(3):622–627. doi:10.1016/j.appet.2008.04.271
4. Dhillon J, Lee JY, Mattes RD. The cephalic phase insulin response to nutritive and low-calorie sweeteners in solid and beverage form. *Physiol Behav.* 2017;181:100–109. doi:10.1016/J.PHYSBEH.2017.09.009
5. Teff KL, Mattes RD, Engelman K, Mattern J. Cephalic-phase insulin in obese and normal-weight men: Relation to postprandial insulin. *Metabolism.* 1993;42(12):1600–1608. doi:10.1016/0026-0495(93)90157-J
6. Tonosaki, Hori, Shimizu, Tonosaki. Relationships between insulin release and taste.
7. Glynn EL, Fry CS, Drummond MJ, et al. Excess leucine intake enhances muscle anabolic signaling but not net protein anabolism in young men and women. *J Nutr.* 2010;140(11):1970–1976. doi:10.3945/jn.110.127647

5: KEEP IT CLEAN! LEARN HOW WE FAST CLEAN

1. Tonosaki K, Hori Y, Shimizu Y, Tonosaki K. Relationships between insulin release and taste. *Biomed Res.* 2007;28(2):79–83.
2. Pietrocola F, Malik SA, Mariño G, et al. Coffee induces autophagy in vivo. *Cell Cycle.* 2014;13(12):1987–1994. doi:10.4161/cc.28929
3. Ryu S, Choi SK, Joung SS, et al. Caffeine as a lipolytic food component increases endurance performance in rats and athletes. *J Nutr Sci Vitaminol (Tokyo).* 2001;47(2):139–146.
4. Martin JV, Nolan B, Wagner GC, Fisher H. Effects of dietary caffeine and alcohol on liver carbohydrate and fat metabolism in rats. *Med Sci Monit.* 2004;10(12):BR455–461.

5. Xie X, Yi W, Zhang P, et al. Green tea polyphenols, mimicking the effects of dietary restriction, ameliorate high-fat diet-induced kidney injury via regulating autophagy flux. *Nutrients*. 2017;9(5). doi:10.3390/nu9050497

6. Finnell JS, Saul BC, Goldhamer AC, Myers TR. Is fasting safe? A chart review of adverse events during medically supervised, water-only fasting. *BMC Complement Altern Med*. 2018;18(1):67. doi:10.1186/s12906-018-2136-6

6: TIME-RESTRICTED EATING:
AN "EATING WINDOW" APPROACH

1. Klein S, Sakurai Y, Romijn JA, Carroll RM. Progressive alterations in lipid and glucose metabolism during short-term fasting in young adult men. *Am J Physiol*. 1993;265(5 Pt 1):E801–E806. doi:10.1152/ajpendo.1993.265.5.E801

2. Stote KS, Baer DJ, Spears K, et al. A controlled trial of reduced meal frequency without caloric restriction in healthy, normal-weight, middle-aged adults. *Am J Clin Nutr*. 2007;85(4):981–988. doi:10.1093/ajcn/85.4.981

3. Van Norren K, Rusli F, Van Dijk M, et al. Behavioural changes are a major contributing factor in the reduction of sarcopenia in caloric-restricted ageing mice. 2015. doi:10.1002/jcsm.12024

4. Acosta-Rodríguez VA, De Groot MHM, Rijo-Ferreira F, Green CB, Takahashi JS. Mice under caloric restriction self-impose a temporal restriction of food intake as revealed by an automated feeder system. *Cell Metab*. 2017;26:267–277. doi:10.1016/j.cmet.2017.06.007

5. Davoodi SH, Ajami M, Ayatollahi SA, Dowlatshahi K, Javedan G, Pazoki-Toroudi HR. Calorie shifting diet versus calorie restriction diet: A comparative clinical trial study. *Int J Prev Med*. 2014;5(4):447–456.

6. Ibid.

7. Sutton EF, Beyl R, Early KS, Cefalu WT, Ravussin E, Peterson CM. Early time-restricted feeding improves insulin sensitivity, blood pressure, and oxidative stress even without weight loss in men with prediabetes. *Cell Metab*. 2018;27. doi:10.1016/j.cmet.2018.04.010

8. Hutchison AT, Regmi P, Manoogian ENC, et al. Time-restricted feeding improves glucose tolerance in men at risk for type 2 diabetes: A randomized crossover trial. *Obesity*. 2019;27(5):oby.22449. doi:10.1002/oby.22449

9. Ibid.

7: ALTERNATE-DAY FASTING PROTOCOLS: THE "UP-AND-DOWN-DAY" APPROACH

1. Davoodi SH, Ajami M, Ayatollahi SA, Dowlatshahi K, Javedan G, Pazoki-Toroudi HR. Calorie shifting diet versus calorie restriction diet: A comparative clinical trial study. *Int J Prev Med.* 2014;5(4):447–456.
2. Dirlewanger M, di Vetta V, Guenat E, et al. Effects of short-term carbohydrate or fat overfeeding on energy expenditure and plasma leptin concentrations in healthy female subjects. *Int J Obes Relat Metab Disord.* 2000;24(11):1413–1418.
3. Harris AM, Jensen MD, Levine JA. Weekly changes in basal metabolic rate with eight weeks of overfeeding. *Obesity.* 2006;14(4):690–695. doi:10.1038/oby.2006.78
4. Varady KA. Intermittent versus daily calorie restriction: Which diet regimen is more effective for weight loss? *Obes Rev.* 2011;12(7):e593–e601. doi:10.1111/j.1467-789X.2011.00873.x
5. Alhamdan BA, Garcia-Alvarez A, Alzahrnai AH, et al. Alternate-day versus daily energy restriction diets: Which is more effective for weight loss? A systematic review and meta-analysis. *Obes Sci Pract.* 2016;2(3):293–302. doi:10.1002/osp4.52

8: YOUR INTERMITTENT FASTING TOOLBOX

1. Keesey RE, Hirvonen MD. Body weight set-points: Determination and adjustment. *J Nutr.* 1997;127(9):1875S–1883S. doi:10.1093/jn/127.9.1875S
2. Iepsen EW, Lundgren J, Holst JJ, Madsbad S, Torekov SS. Successful weight loss maintenance includes long-term increased meal responses of GLP-1 and PYY3–36. *Eur J Endocrinol.* 2016;174(6):775–784. doi:10.1530/EJE-15-1116
3. Davoodi SH, Ajami M, Ayatollahi SA, Dowlatshahi K, Javedan G, Pazoki-Toroudi HR. Calorie shifting diet versus calorie restriction diet: A comparative clinical trial study. *Int J Prev Med.* 2014;5(4):447–456.

9: JUST SAY NO: FASTING RED FLAGS

1. Janse van Rensburg D, Nolte K. Sports injuries in adults: Overview of clinical examination and management. *South African Fam Pract.* 2011;53(1):21–27. doi:10.1080/20786204.2011.10874055
2. Webber J, Macdonald IA. The cardiovascular, metabolic and hormonal changes accompanying acute starvation in men and women. *Br J Nutr.* 1994;71(3):437–447.
3. (UK) NCC for MH. Diagnostic criteria for eating disorders. 2004.
4. Hoddy KK, Kroeger CM, Trepanowski JF, Barnosky AR, Bhutani S, Varady KA. Safety of alternate day fasting and effect on disordered eating behaviors. *Nutr J.* 2015;14. doi:10.1186/s12937-015-0029-9

5. Childhood Obesity Facts | Healthy Schools | CDC. https://www.cdc.gov /healthyschools/obesity/facts.htm. Accessed July 30, 2019.
6. Ramadan Fast: Should Children Give Up Food and Water? - BBC News. https://www.bbc.com/news/world-europe-44107950. Accessed July 30, 2019.
7. Riordan J. Breastfeeding and Human Lactation - Jan Riordan - Google Books. https://books.google.com/books?id=aiVesab_2bwC&printsec=frontcover&dq =Breastfeeding+and+Human+Lactation+riordan&hl=en&sa=X&ved= 0ahUKEwieyaX_xt3jAhWJneAKHZ_iBO0Q6AEIKDAA#v=onepage&q =Breastfeeding and Human Lactation riordan&f=false. Accessed July 30, 2019.

13: "DIET BRAIN" AND HOW TO AVOID IT

1. Yamagishi K, Iso H, Yatsuya H, et al. Dietary intake of saturated fatty acids and mortality from cardiovascular disease in Japanese: The Japan Collaborative Cohort Study for Evaluation of Cancer Risk (JACC) Study. *Am J Clin Nutr.* 2010;92(4):759–765. doi:10.3945/ajcn.2009.29146
2. Kitada M, Ogura Y, Monno I, Koya D. The impact of dietary protein intake on longevity and metabolic health. *EBioMedicine.* 2019;43:632–640. doi:10.1016/j. ebiom.2019.04.005

14: BIO-INDIVIDUALITY

1. What Is the Best Diet for Humans? | Eran Segal | TEDxRuppin - YouTube. https://www.youtube.com/watch?v=0z03xkwFbw4. Accessed July 31, 2019.
2. Zeevi D, Korem T, Zmora N, et al. Personalized nutrition by prediction of glycemic responses article personalized nutrition by prediction of glycemic responses. *Cell.* 2015;163:1079–1094. doi:10.1016/j.cell.2015.11.001
3. About Glycemic Index. http://www.glycemicindex.com/about.php. Accessed August 1, 2019.
4. Glycemic Index for 60+ Foods - Harvard Health. https://www.health.harvard .edu/diseases-and-conditions/glycemic-index-and-glycemic-load-for-100 -foods. Accessed August 1, 2019.
5. *Overview of the ZOE Scientific Project for Researchers & Clinicians;* 2019.
6. Spector T, et al. Predicting personal metabolic responses to food using multi-omics machine learning in over 1000 twins and singletons from the UK and US: The PREDICT 1 Study. *Curr Dev Nutr.* 2019;3(Suppl 1):nzz037. doi:10.1093/cdn/nzz037.OR31-01-19
7. Hamideh D, Arellano B, Topol EJ, Steinhubl SR. Your digital nutritionist. *Lancet (London, England).* 2019;393(10166):19. doi:10.1016/S0140-6736(18)33170-2

8. Fumagalli M, Camus SM, Diekmann Y, et al. Genetic diversity of CHC22 clathrin impacts its function in glucose metabolism. *Elife.* 2019;8. doi:10.7554/eLife.41517

15: THE END OF THE CALORIE

1. Hargrove JL. Does the history of food energy units suggest a solution to "calorie confusion"? *Nutr J.* 2007;6:44. doi:10.1186/1475-2891-6-44
2. Carmody RN, Weintraub GS, Wrangham RW. Energetic consequences of thermal and nonthermal food processing. *Proc Natl Acad Sci USA.* 2011;108(48):19199–19203. doi:10.1073/pnas.1112128108
3. Barr SB, Wright JC. Postprandial energy expenditure in whole-food and processed-food meals: Implications for daily energy expenditure. *Food Nutr Res.* 2010;54. doi:10.3402/fnr.v54i0.5144
4. Groopman EE, Carmody RN, Wrangham RW. Cooking increases net energy gain from a lipid-rich food. *Am J Phys Anthropol.* 2015;156(1):11–18. doi:10.1002/ajpa.22622
5. Novotny JA, Gebauer SK, Baer DJ. Discrepancy between the Atwater factor predicted and empirically measured energy values of almonds in human diets. *Am J Clin Nutr.* 2012;96(2):296–301. doi:10.3945/ajcn.112.035782
6. Baer DJ, Gebauer SK, Novotny JA. Walnuts consumed by healthy adults provide less available energy than predicted by the Atwater factors. *J Nutr.* 2016;146(1):9–13. doi:10.3945/jn.115.217372
7. Horton TJ, Drougas H, Brachey A, Reed GW, Peters JC, Hill JO. Fat and carbohydrate overfeeding in humans: Different effects on energy storage. *Am J Clin Nutr.* 1995;62(1):19–29. doi:10.1093/ajcn/62.1.19
8. Dirlewanger M, di Vetta V, Guenat E, et al. Effects of short-term carbohydrate or fat overfeeding on energy expenditure and plasma leptin concentrations in healthy female subjects. *Int J Obes Relat Metab Disord.* 2000;24(11):1413–1418.

16: APPETITE CORRECTION:
WHAT EXACTLY IS THIS HORMONAL VOODOO?

1. Intuitive Eating. https://www.intuitiveeating.org/. Accessed August 5, 2019.
2. Gruzdeva O, Borodkina D, Uchasova E, Dyleva Y, Barbarash O. Leptin resistance: Underlying mechanisms and diagnosis. *Diabetes Metab Syndr Obes.* 2019;12:191–198. doi:10.2147/DMSO.S182406

3. *From Lesions to Leptin: Review Hypothalamic Control of Food Intake and Body Weight.*

4. Erlanson-Albertsson C. How palatable food disrupts appetite regulation. *Basic Clin Pharmacol Toxicol.* 2005;97(2):61–73. doi:10.1111/j.1742-7843.2005. pto_179.x

5. Tremblay A, Royer M-M, Chaput J-P, Doucet É. Adaptive thermogenesis can make a difference in the ability of obese individuals to lose body weight. *Int J Obes.* 2013;37:759–764. doi:10.1038/ijo.2012.124

6. Ravussin E, Beyl RA, Poggiogalle E, Hsia DS, Peterson CM. Early time-restricted feeding reduces appetite and increases fat oxidation but does not affect energy expenditure in humans. *Obesity.* 2019;27(8):1244–1254. doi:10.1002/oby.22518

7. Ahima RS, Antwi DA. Brain regulation of appetite and satiety. *Endocrinol Metab Clin North Am.* 2008;37(4):811–823. doi:10.1016/j.ecl.2008.08.005

8. Tremblay, Royer, Chaput, Doucet. Adaptive thermogenesis can make a difference.

17: BEANS VERSUS JELLY BEANS:
DOES FOOD QUALITY MATTER?

1. Augusto Monteiro C, Cannon G, Moubarac J-C, Bertazzi Levy R, Laura Louzada MC, Constante Jaime P. The UN Decade of Nutrition, the NOVA food classification and the trouble with ultra-processing. 2017. doi:10.1017/S1368980017000234

2. Ibid.

3. *Food Systems and Diets: Facing the Challenges of the 21st Century;* 2016.

4. Monteiro CA, Cannon G, Levy RB, et al. Ultra-processed foods: What they are and how to identify them. *Public Health Nutr.* 2019;22(5):936–941. doi:10.1017/S1368980018003762

5. *Food Systems and Diets.*

6. Hall KD, Ayuketah A, Brychta R, et al. Ultra-processed diets cause excess calorie intake and weight gain: An inpatient randomized controlled trial of ad libitum food intake. *Cell Metab.* 2019;30(1):67–77.e3. doi:10.1016/J.CMET.2019.05.008

7. Ibid.

8. de Macedo IC, de Freitas JS, da Silva Torres IL. The influence of palatable diets in reward system activation: A mini review. *Adv Pharmacol Sci.* 2016;2016:7238679. doi:10.1155/2016/7238679

18: SCALE-SCHMALE:
THE ULTIMATE GUIDE TO TRACKING YOUR PROGRESS

1. Ashwell M, Mayhew L, Richardson J, Rickayzen B. Waist-to-height ratio is more predictive of years of life lost than body mass index. *PLOS ONE.* 2014;9(9): e103483. doi:10.1371/journal.pone.0103483
2. Murray S. Is waist-to-hip ratio a better marker of cardiovascular risk than body mass index? *CMAJ.* 2006;174(3):308. doi:10.1503/cmaj.051561

20: GET YOUR MIND RIGHT!

1. Tétreault P, Mansour A, Vachon-Presseau E, Schnitzer TJ, Apkarian AV, Baliki MN. Brain connectivity predicts placebo response across chronic pain clinical trials. Wager TD, ed. *PLOS Biol.* 2016;14(10):e1002570. doi:10.1371/journal.pbio.1002570
2. Crum AJ, Langer EJ. Mindset matters: Exercise and the placebo effect. *Psychol Sci.* 2007;18(2):165–171. doi:10.1111/j.1467-9280.2007.01867.x
3. Hoffmann V, Lanz M, Mackert J, Müller T, Tschöp M, Meissner K. Effects of placebo interventions on subjective and objective markers of appetite—A randomized controlled trial. *Front Psychiatry.* 2018;9:706. doi:10.3389/fpsyt.2018.00706
4. Panayotov VS. Studying a possible placebo effect of an imaginary low-calorie diet. *Front Psychiatry.* 2019;10:550. doi:10.3389/fpsyt.2019.00550
5. Ranganathan VK, Siemionow V, Liu JZ, Sahgal V, Yue GH. From mental power to muscle power—gaining strength by using the mind. *Neuropsychologia.* 2004;42(7):944–956. doi:10.1016/j.neuropsychologia.2003.11.018
6. Levy BR, Slade MD, Kunkel SR, Kasl SV. Longevity increased by positive self-perceptions of aging. *J Pers Soc Psychol.* 2002;83(2):261–270.
7. Maruta T, Colligan RC, Malinchoc M, Offord KP. Optimism-pessimism assessed in the 1960s and self-reported health status 30 years later. *Mayo Clin Proc.* 2002;77(8):748–753. doi:10.4065/77.8.748
8. Maruta T, Colligan RC, Malinchoc M, Offord KP. Optimists vs pessimists: Survival rate among medical patients over a 30-year period. *Mayo Clin Proc.* 2000;75(2):140–143. doi:10.4065/75.2.140
9. Hernandez R, Kershaw KN, Siddique J, et al. Optimism and cardiovascular health: Multi-Ethnic Study of Atherosclerosis (MESA). *Heal Behav Policy Rev.* 2015;2(1):62–73. doi:10.14485/HBPR.2.1.6

21: GET MOVING! FAST-FUELED FITNESS

1. Swift DL, Johannsen NM, Lavie CJ, Earnest CP, Church TS. The role of exercise and physical activity in weight loss and maintenance. *Prog Cardiovasc Dis.* 2014;56(4):441–447. doi:10.1016/j.pcad.2013.09.012
2. Lee I-M, Hsieh C, Paffenbarger RS. Exercise intensity and longevity in Men. *JAMA.* 1995;273(15):1179. doi:10.1001/jama.1995.03520390039030
3. Warburton DER, Nicol CW, Bredin SSD. Health benefits of physical activity: The evidence. *CMAJ.* 2006;174(6):801–809. doi:10.1503/cmaj.051351
4. Dunn AL, Trivedi MH, O'Neal HA. Physical activity dose-response effects on outcomes of depression and anxiety. *Med Sci Sports Exerc.* 2001;33(6 Suppl): S587–S97; discussion 609–610.
5. LaMonte MJ, Buchner DM, Rillamas-Sun E, et al. Accelerometer-measured physical activity and mortality in women aged 63 to 99. *J Am Geriatr Soc.* 2018;66(5):886–894. doi:10.1111/jgs.15201
6. LaCroix AZ, Bellettiere J, Rillamas-Sun E, et al. Association of light physical activity measured by accelerometry and incidence of coronary heart disease and cardiovascular disease in older women. *JAMA Netw Open.* 2019;2(3):e190419. doi:10.1001/jamanetworkopen.2019.0419
7. Jones N, Kiely J, Suraci B, et al. A genetic-based algorithm for personalized resistance-training. *Biol Sport.* 2016;33(2):117–126. doi:10.5604/20831862.1198210
8. Møller AB, Vendelbo MH, Christensen B, et al. Physical exercise increases autophagic signaling through ULK1 in human skeletal muscle. *J Appl Physiol.* 2015;118(8):971–979. doi:10.1152/japplphysiol.01116.2014
9. Anton SD, Moehl K, Donahoo WT, et al. Flipping the metabolic switch: Understanding and applying the health benefits of fasting. *Obesity (Silver Spring).* 2018;26(2):254–268. doi:10.1002/oby.22065
10. Ibid.
11. Schoenfeld BJ, Aragon AA, Krieger JW. The effect of protein timing on muscle strength and hypertrophy: A meta-analysis. *J Int Soc Sports Nutr.* 2013;10(1):53. doi:10.1186/1550-2783-10-53
12. Salgin B, Marcovecchio ML, Hill N, Dunger DB, Frystyk J. The effect of prolonged fasting on levels of growth hormone–binding protein and free growth hormone. *Growth Horm IGF Res.* 2012;22(2):76–81. doi:10.1016/j. ghir.2012.02.003
13. Ho KY, Veldhuis JD, Johnson ML, et al. Fasting enhances growth hormone secretion and amplifies the complex rhythms of growth hormone secretion in man. *J Clin Invest.* 1988;81(4):968–975. doi:10.1172/JCI113450
14. Graham TE. Caffeine and exercise: Metabolism, endurance, and performance. *Sport Med.* 2001;31(11):785-807. doi:10.2165/00007256-200131110-00002
15. Teruya T, Chaleckis R, Takada J, Yanagida M, Kondoh H. Diverse metabolic reactions activated during 58-hr fasting are revealed by non-targeted

metabolomic analysis of human blood. *Sci Rep.* 2019;9(1):854. doi:10.1038/s41598-018-36674-9

16. Bröer S, Bröer A. Amino acid homeostasis and signalling in mammalian cells and organisms. *Biochem J.* 2017;474(12):1935–1963. doi:10.1042/BCJ20160822

17. Sou Y, Waguri S, Iwata J, et al. The Atg8 conjugation system is indispensable for proper development of autophagic isolation membranes in mice. Subramani S, ed. *Mol Biol Cell.* 2008;19(11):4762–4775. doi:10.1091/mbc.e08-03-0309

22: WEIGHT LOSS TOO SLOW OR YOU'RE AT A PLATEAU? HOW TO ADJUST AND ADAPT

1. Shelmet JJ, Reichard GA, Skutches CL, Hoeldtke RD, Owen OE, Boden G. Ethanol causes acute inhibition of carbohydrate, fat, and protein oxidation and insulin resistance. *J Clin Invest.* 1988;81(4):1137–1145. doi:10.1172/JCI113428

2. Siler SQ, Neese RA, Hellerstein MK. De novo lipogenesis, lipid kinetics, and whole-body lipid balances in humans after acute alcohol consumption. *Am J Clin Nutr.* 1999;70(5):928–936. doi:10.1093/ajcn/70.5.928

3. Yeomans MR. Short term effects of alcohol on appetite in humans. Effects of context and restrained eating. *Appetite.* 2010;55(3):565–573. doi:10.1016/J.APPET.2010.09.005

24: SHARE WITHOUT FEAR

1. Foodinsight.org. *2018 Food & Health Survey;* 2018.

FREQUENTLY ASKED QUESTIONS

1. Arnason TG, Bowen MW, Mansell KD. Effects of intermittent fasting on health markers in those with type 2 diabetes: A pilot study. *World J Diabetes.* 2017;8(4):154–164. doi:10.4239/wjd.v8.i4.154

2. Furmli S, Elmasry R, Ramos M, Fung J. Therapeutic use of intermittent fasting for people with type 2 diabetes as an alternative to insulin. *BMJ Case Rep.* 2018;2018. doi:10.1136/bcr-2017-221854

3. Soules MR, Merriggiola MC, Steiner RA, Clifton DK, Toivola B, Bremner WJ. Short-term fasting in normal women: Absence of effects on gonadotrophin secretion and the menstrual cycle. *Clin Endocrinol (Oxford).* 1994;40(6):725–731.

4. Nair PMK, Khawale PG. Role of therapeutic fasting in women's health: An overview. *J Midlife Health*. 2016;7(2):61–64. doi:10.4103/0976-7800.185325

5. Wang A, Huen SC, Luan HH, et al. Opposing effects of fasting metabolism on tissue tolerance in bacterial and viral inflammation. *Cell*. 2016;166(6):1512–1525.e12. doi:10.1016/j.cell.2016.07.026

6. Pietrocola F, Malik SA, Mariño G, et al. Coffee induces autophagy in vivo. *Cell Cycle*. 2014;13(12):1987–1994. doi:10.4161/cc.28929

7. Cigarette Ingredients: R.J. Reynolds Tobacco Company. https://www.rjrt.com /commercial-integrity/ingredients/cigarette-ingredients/. Accessed July 5, 2019.

8. Bajaj M. Nicotine and insulin resistance: When the smoke clears. *Diabetes*. 2012;61(12):3078–3080. doi:10.2337/db12-1100

9. Attvall S, Fowelin J, Lager I, Von Schenck H, Smith U. Smoking induces insulin resistance—A potential link with the insulin resistance syndrome. *J Intern Med*. 1993;233(4):327–332.

10. Tapsell LC, Neale EP, Satija A, Hu FB. Foods, nutrients, and dietary patterns: Interconnections and implications for dietary guidelines. *Adv Nutr*. 2016;7(3): 445–454. doi:10.3945/an.115.011718

11. Olsson K-E, Saltin B. Variation in total body water with muscle glycogen changes in man. *Acta Physiol Scand*. 1970;80(1):11–18. doi:10.1111/j.1748-1716 .1970.tb04764.x

12. Zangeneh F, Abedinia N, Mehdi Naghizadeh M, Salman Yazdi R, Madani T. The effect of Ramadan fasting on hypothalamic pituitary ovarian (HPO) axis in women with polycystic ovary syndrome. *Women's Heal Bull*. 2014;1(1). doi:10.17795/whb-18962

13. Marshall JC, Dunaif A. Should all women with PCOS be treated for insulin resistance? *Fertil Steril*. 2012;97(1):18–22. doi:10.1016/j.fertnstert.2011.11.036

14. Cho S, Dietrich M, Brown CJP, Clark CA, Block G. *The Effect of Breakfast Type on Total Daily Energy Intake and Body Mass Index: Results from the Third National Health and Nutrition Examination Survey (NHANES III)*.

15. Sievert K, Hussain SM, Page MJ, et al. Effect of breakfast on weight and energy intake: Systematic review and meta-analysis of randomised controlled trials. *BMJ*. 2019;364:l42. doi:10.1136/bmj.l42

16. Anton SD, Moehl K, Donahoo WT, et al. Flipping the metabolic switch: Understanding and applying the health benefits of fasting. *Obesity (Silver Spring)*. 2018;26(2):254–268. doi:10.1002/oby.22065

17. Funada J, Dennis AL, Roberts R, Karpe F, Frayn KN. Regulation of subcutaneous adipose tissue blood flow is related to measures of vascular and autonomic function. *Clin Sci*. 2010;119(8):313–322. doi:10.1042/CS20100066

18. Landsberg L, Young JB, Leonard WR, Linsenmeier RA, Turek FW. Do the obese have lower body temperatures? A new look at a forgotten variable in energy balance. *Trans Am Clin Climatol Assoc*. 2009;120:287–295.

19. Phinney SD, Tang AB, Waggoner CR, Tezanos-Pinto RG, Davis PA. The transient hypercholesterolemia of major weight loss. *Am J Clin Nutr*. 1991;53(6): 1404–1410. doi:10.1093/ajcn/53.6.1404

INDEX

Franken-foods, 2, 3
free radicals, 46
frequently asked questions, 271–308
frontal lobes, 216
fructose, as insulin trigger, 20
fuel sources
    autophagy, 39–43
    fat stores, 16, 18, 23–27, 42–43, 48–49,
        53, 58–60, 82, 85, 97, 114, 122–24,
        223–24, 296
    glycogen stores, 17–18, 20–21, 23–24,
        121–22, 142, 225, 298, 308
    metabolic flexibility and, 25
    multiple, in metabolic adaptation, 16
    subcutaneous/visceral fat, 36–37, 302
Fuhrman, Joel, 110
Fung, Jason, 31–32, 41, 276, 277–78, 289,
    291, 299

genetic factors
    DNA analysis, 2–3, 159–60, 221–22
    in glucose response, 157
Georgia State University, 48
ghrelin (hunger hormone)
    in appetite correction, 7, 169–76
    increase in, 9–10, 217
    intermittent fasting and, 11, 37–38,
        102, 123
Global Panel on Agriculture and Food
    Systems for Nutrition, 180
glucagon, 17–18
glucagon-like peptide 1, 173
gluconeogenesis, 45
glycemic index (GI), 154–56
glycemic response, 66
glycogen, 63
    depleting stores of, 17–18, 20–21, 23–24,
        121–22, 142, 225, 298, 308
    in FAST Start, 121–22
    refilling stores of, 207
goal weight/goal body, 2, 143–44, 153, 158,
    239–42
Grain Brain (Perlmutter), 149
growth mindset, 211–12
gum, chewing, 54, 55, 57, 62, 66, 209–10,
    231, 294
gut microbiome, 38, 156–60, 166, 221,
    298

hair loss, 299
Happy Scale app, 193
hara hachi bu, 174
Harvard University, 48
Hashimoto's thyroiditis, 34
headache, 65, 121

heart disease, 18, 30, 31, 33, 35, 48, 155,
    198, 220, 302
Heller, Rachael F., 2
Heller, Richard F., 2
herbal tea, 57, 62, 68
Herring, Bert, 85–86, 170–73, 208–9
hippocampus, 36
homeostasis
    impact of, 101–3
    switching things up, 103–7, 134–35,
        232–33
honesty pants, 199, 200, 230–31, 242–44
honey, 55
hormone injections, 3
human growth hormone (HGH), 26–27,
    190–92, 224
hunger
    appetite correction and, 3, 10, 37–38,
        168, 169–76, 184–85, 204, 286, 296
    Delay, Don't Deny approach to, 280–81,
        286
    in FAST Start, 122–23
    internal signals of, 168, 169–70, 174–75,
        281, 292
    in metabolic adaptation, 174–75
    see also ghrelin (hunger hormone)
Huntington's disease, 36
hyperinsulinemia, 18–19, 30, 39, 300
hypothalamus, 171, 173
hypothyroidism, 230, 237

ice cream, 142, 155, 156, 179
immune system
    autoimmune disease, 33, 34–35
    gut microbiome, 38, 156–60, 166, 221, 298
    inflammation and, 33–35
infants
    breastfeeding, 114–15, 278
    human growth hormone (HGH)
        production, 27
    natural appetite control, 37–38, 171, 288
infertility, 229, 278, 300
inflammation, 33–35
inflammatory bowel disease, 33, 34
"inner toddler," 144, 210–11
insulin, 16–27
    antilypolitic effects, 19, 20, 26, 27, 54
    cephalic phase insulin release (CPIR),
        17–18, 54–58, 289, 293, 294
    clean fast levels, 53–58
    hyperinsulinemia, 18–19, 30, 39, 300
    intermittent fasting and, 19–27
    role in body, 17–18
    sweet taste and, 18, 54–58. see also
        sweet taste